The Ultimate Guide to Bodyweight Squats and Pistols

2nd Edition

By Logan Christopher

DISCLAIMER

The exercises and training information contained within this book may be too strenuous or dangerous for some people, and the reader should consult with a physician before engaging in them. The health advice contained within this book is for educational purposes only and is not intended for medical purposes.

The author and publisher of this book are not responsible in any manner whatsoever for the use, misuse or dis-use of the information presented here.

Published by:

Legendary Strength LLC

Santa Cruz, California

www.LegendaryStrength.com

Table of Contents

Introduction to this Book and the Series

The Ultimate Guide to Bodyweight Squats and Pistols is all about exactly what the title says it is.

This is just one book in a series of five in The Ultimate Guide to Bodyweight Exercises series. The other titles are:

- The Ultimate Guide to Handstand Pushups
- The Ultimate Guide to Pullups and Chin-ups
- The Ultimate Guide to Bodyweight Ab Exercises
- The Ultimate Guide to Bodyweight Conditioning Exercises

And maybe I'll be expanding the series out further in the future. (The Ultimate Guide to Levers and Flags has a nice ring to it.)

The aim of this series is not to make an exhaustive encyclopedia of every possible version and variation that is out there. While there are plenty of variations within these pages, just having those without a clear training path can hinder progress.

Instead, these books are all about walking you through the exact steps, variants and progressions you need to hit a variety of goals. Whether it is hitting your first rep in many classic exercises like a handstand pushup, pullup or pistol squat, or mastering these exercises to an elite level, you'll find what you need inside.

The name of the game in training is progress and how to go from one level to the next is the key aim of each book. If I could go from not being able to do pushups, let alone handstand pushups, or pullups or one-legged squats to what I can do today, then you can too.

I first created The Ultimate Guide to Handstand Pushups back in 2009, almost a decade ago. The other books in the series came between 2013 and 2014. As you might imagine, I've learned a few things since that time, both in my own training and experimentation as well as working with clients. In addition to learning from many others, I've developed techniques and methods that no one else knows about (at least until they read this).

That is why in the newly revamped 2nd editions the title of "Ultimate Guide" becomes even truer. You'll find some stuff in here that simply isn't covered elsewhere.

As exercise technique is not best demonstrated by text and even pictures, each course is accompanied by a complete optional video series. In those you'll find additional material not covered in the books.

If you want to pick up the other books in the series, as well as the accompanying videos, you'll find these all available at https://legendarystrength.com/books-videos/. In addition, you'll find everything else I've created outside of bodyweight training from strongman to kettlebells, health to mental training, all there.

Why the Squat?

The squat is known as the king of exercises. Usually, this refers to the weighted version, the back squat, but that doesn't mean bodyweight squats are any less royal.

A significant portion of the muscle mass of the body is in the legs. The quadriceps, hamstrings and glutes are large muscle groups and must be worked by anyone that wants to be strong and fit.

Because most of the muscle mass is in the legs, this makes various squatting exercises great for conditioning. As you are moving all your bodyweight, can do it quickly, and the big muscles are in use, squats will typically get your lungs going as well. (Up to a point. Very conditioned athletes can often do bodyweight squatting for long periods of time without getting out of breath, one of the subjects of this book.)

A third benefit is that squatting brings flexibility. That is, if you do it in a full range of motion. Because so few people do squats and use this range of motion in their daily life, they LOSE IT! But fear not as it can be reclaimed.

This book is divided into six modules.

The first is all about the basic form of the squat and how to use it to build your flexibility. Goal number one for anyone working with squats is to acquire and maintain a full range of motion. Can you still build strength and endurance without it? Absolutely, but as you improve those capabilities you can work your flexibility at the same time. We'll end this section with what it takes to be able to relax and rest in that rock bottom position.

Module two is all about opening tons of variations of the squat. Many of these are harder than the basic form. Many target certain muscles more than others. Many require additional flexibility beyond the regular squat. These all make good building blocks for the upcoming sections. You'll also find lunges and various jumping squat here too. While you want to get a good handle on the basic squat form in the beginning, you then want to translate that into being able to squat and lunge in a wide variety of ways for greater strength, endurance, flexibility and mobility. Here we'll also focus on starting to build up to moderate rep ranges.

Module three goes on to reveal what it takes to do hundreds or even thousands of reps. This is one possible direction of bodyweight leg training. Having done a thousand reps in a single set of Hindu squats, I have some tips to lend here. These training methods will show you how you can do the same if you choose to pursue these endurance goals.

Module four covers what I once considered the ultimate of bodyweight squats, the pistol or one-legged squat. This beginner section covers details on form and how to work up to your first pistol including many tips, tricks and methods to get there.

In module five, you'll move beyond your first rep and discover how to master the pistol with advanced variations, added resistance, repping out, explosiveness and more.

Finally, in module six we'll cover the other one-legged squat variations including how to work up to your first reps and the more advanced steps to take. These include shrimp squats, figure 4 squats and the dragon pistol. This culminates in what I like to call the 4-Way One Legged Squat challenge.

Throughout this book you'll find lots of detail along with the pictures and training plans for each section. The aim is to give you everything you need technique and training-wise to make forward progress.

Bodyweight versus Weights

At one point in my life I was a "bodyweight only" guy. I was (mis)lead to believe that weights were stupid, non-functional and dangerous. I no longer believe that. Each tool, bodyweight included, has its advantages and drawbacks.

The advantages of bodyweight training are that it requires little to no equipment and can be done pretty much anywhere. When the biggest excuse for people not working out is lack of time or access to a gym, bodyweight training at home is an excellent solution. Furthermore, by working bodyweight people tend to get more in tune with their body than if they just manipulate weights.

Yet, one of the disadvantages of bodyweight is how they hit the lower body. Although I spend a significant portion of my training time with bodyweight exercises you can only go so far with them, at least when it comes to the lower body. The upper body limits are much further out. Until you're cranking out freestanding full range handstand pushups and one arm pull-ups you've still got some distance to go.

Because the leg muscles are stronger, most will be able to work up to pistols within a short amount of time. In fact, for many people it's not a matter of strength, as much as it is of flexibility to do the exercise. Although you can do advanced variations, higher jumps, and many reps it's not always the biggest challenge on your lower body. The other one-legged squat variations amp up flexibility demands even more so.

Exercises like deadlifts, front and back squats have their place. Among circus professionals and gymnasts, you won't see many feats requiring the strongest legs. Some strength is certainly needed for various acrobatics. But all the most amazing skills of these athletes utilize upper body strength.

I'm not saying you can't stick to bodyweight only if you choose to. I just want to make you aware of this fact. Along with that, I will feature some weights in this book. Since this is a book about bodyweight squats and not weighted squats, its limited. Still, these weights can be used in a variety of ways to increase what you can accomplish.

You may choose to focus on bodyweight exercises with the upper body and weights for the lower body. I've done this at times myself and know others who have as well. And then there are other times where I was solely focused on bodyweight leg training. Cycling between weighted work and bodyweight work is something I've been doing for years and find works well for keeping up my interest and well-roundedness.

The Keys of Progression (especially for Bodyweight)

The fact is, if you don't have progress built in, then you're likely just spinning your wheels, like a hamster in a cage. That's why they call it progressive strength training. Or progressive conditioning.

The lack of clear and effective progression is the failing of most fitness programs.

With weights it's simple. Just get more weight on the bar or lift a heavier kettlebell. That is one form of progress. Unfortunately, simply going after that will only get you so far.

When it comes to bodyweight training, you can't simply remove or add weight! This means that you must use a variety of other factors to ensure progress in intensity happens. These include, but are not limited to, changes in range of motion, changes in leverage, tightening up form, and going from two limbs to one.

In many bodyweight training programs, the steps between exercises are too big. I'll pick on *Convict Conditioning*. Overall, it's an amazing book and the sequels are great too. I've communicated with Paul Wade (he even wrote the forward to my book *Mental Muscle*), so I don't mean disrespect. But in having ten steps for each progression you'll find that in some the jump from one step to the next is tiny. It's easy and most people could make that progress essentially from one workout to the next. Yet in other cases the steps are a massive jump, where a year of training on the previous step still might not get you there. Showing just ten steps is great for simplicity yet breaks down in effectiveness.

I'm going to ask you think a little bit more. You must be smart about your progress. And it's in working on bodyweight exercises coming up on two decades now that I've figured out steps that many other people miss. Understand the ideas behind the exercises and progressions laid out here and you'll be able to take this foundation into anything you do.

Here's an example. I'm often asked about one of my most famous feats of strength, pulling an 8,800 lb. fire truck with my hair. How did I accomplish that? Progressive strength training. I started with smaller vehicles that I could pull. I work on doing some longer distances. Then I started working with bigger vehicles (from a truck, to a fifteen-passenger van loaded with band equipment, to an RV). I worked going slightly uphill with some of these. It's the same principles of progress behind this as it is behind any form of training, bodyweight included.

In the following pages, the bodyweight exercises are broken up over different modules. These modules are targeted towards where you are at and the goals you're going after. At the end are sample training plans. These can be used as is, or better yet, modified to suit you better.

I'm a huge proponent of learning how to listen to your body. Yes, there is a process behind doing that, which I lay out in *Beyond Biofeedback: The 4 Levels of Intuitive Training*. Following a training plan, come hell or high water is a good way to injure yourself. But in taking the ideas from it, and then modifying based on your body's feedback, you will move forward more safely.

So far, we've only talked about "intensity" as a measure of progress. In weightlifting terms, this means the percentage of your one rep max, in how much weight you're lifting. If we generalize it just a little bit, it is described as the difficulty of an exercise for you. A one-legged squat is more intense than a two-legged squat. A close leg squat is more intense than the basic two-legged squat, but not the pistol.

The other factors at play for progression are volume and density. Volume is the amount of work you do on an exercise which typically comes down to sets and reps. (And in the case of holds, the duration or time.)

Density is the amount of work done in a period of time. This is an important factor in relation to volume, because if you only ever did more, but taking a longer time to do it, you haven't necessarily made progress.

How to use these different measures of progress are laid out in the pages to come. You'll see that it is these, and almost exclusively these, that are what determine your progress. There are a few other progressive factors, such as frequency, but those are of lesser importance. Still they can be very useful at certain times.

I offer this basic primer on progression before we get started to help you to understand what is behind the layout of the modules and exercises to come. For those that want more, the keys to progression are covered in even more detail inside my other book, *The Master Keys to Strength and Fitness*. If you'd like to go deeper to really understand the number one principle behind effective training, I consider that must-read material. And it covers many other foundational concepts to strength and fitness too.

Module 1 - Achieving Full Range of Motion in the Squat

The first goal of this book is to get you into a full range of motion on your squat. In many parts of the world that aren't "Westernized," it's common for people to eat, play and otherwise spend time in the bottom of a squat position. If you don't have a chair it's a great option.

But because many people sit all the time, and never go beyond that parallel level of their legs, they can lose their natural ability. And it is natural. Kids will easily and effortlessly get into this position. It really must be trained out of you through neglect of using it.

But not to worry. It's quite easy to regain this flexibility in time. And it won't require any stretching to do so either, although that can help. We will be working with where you're at and building from there. If you work within your limitations, but near the edge of them, they will expand. And it doesn't have to be hard work either. Simply squat more and you'll get better at squatting.

Of course, there are specific tips and tricks we can use to assist along the way and make the progress faster and easier.

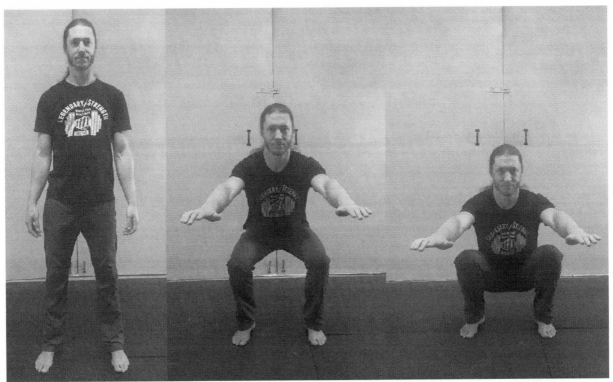

The basic bodyweight squat from the front position.

Squat Form

Stand with the feet shoulder width apart. Some people will be more comfortable a little closer together and others a little wider. There are some specific squat variations we'll be working with later that are very narrow and very wide. For now, shoulder width or just outside it will usually be best. This gives you enough space to open up the hips. Many people end up having their feet too narrow which stops them from descending further down.

While there may be an ideal form you really have to work to find what suits your body. Different people have different limb lengths. Your tibia to your femur to your spine ratio will, in some small part, change what is ideal for you when it comes to squats.

The feet can be pointed straight ahead or just slightly outside. What does straight ahead mean? It can be confusing because it depends on which part of the foot you're looking at to point straight. Use the second toe, the one closest to the big toe, to point straight. Or it can even be more turned outside of that.

Here again, most people will find turning the feet slightly to the outside will assist in doing the squat. Here you may line up the inside edges of your feet to make them parallel, while the second toes are pointed slightly to the outside.

Make sure your heels stay firmly planted on the floor. The basic squat is flat-footed. Coming up on the toes will be covered later and is a different variation. Doing so changes up the mechanics, which muscles are emphasized, and lowers the flexibility needed.

Now that you have your starting position sit back and down until your thighs are resting on your calves. The back should be kept mostly straight (more details on this in a bit). The hands and arms usually come forward to counterbalance your weight.

The test of your squat is can you get into this bottom position and rest there comfortably? If you can, great! Now you'll be adding reps and variations to build your leg power. If not, keep reading for much more detail.

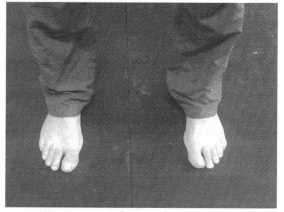 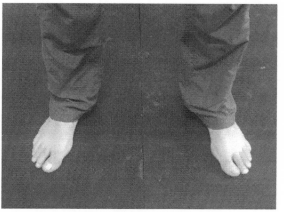

Toes pointed straight ahead and toes to the outside with a slightly wider stance.
Most people will squat easier with the second position.

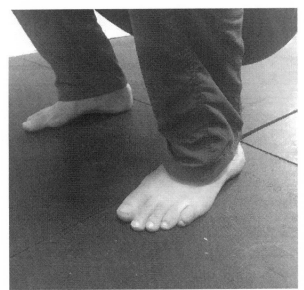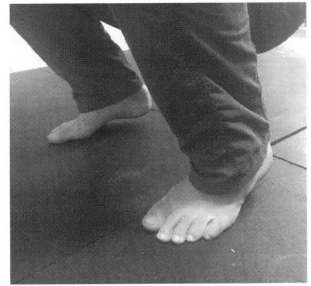

The first picture shows heels firmly on the floor.
Meanwhile, in the second I've raised up onto the toes, which you want to avoid.

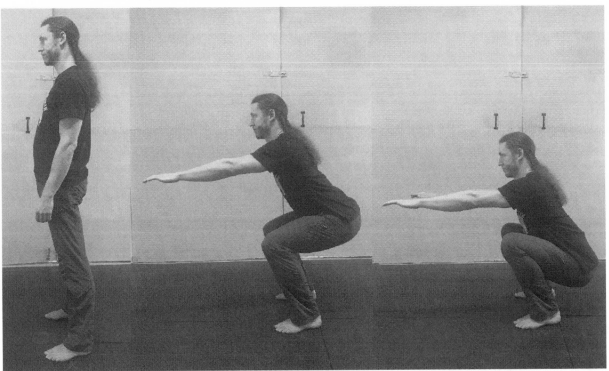

The squat shown from the side shows the basic foot, hip and back position.

Squat Breathing

For bodyweight squats, the breathing typically takes on what is known as anatomical breathing. That is as you squat down you exhale and as you raise up you inhale. This is the natural breathing method for the squat because as you squat down your torso will have less room for the lungs. When you stand up you're expanded, so the lungs have more room.

If you're starting out and feel you need more stability you can breathe in as you lower down. This can help to create pressure in your torso which will allow you to be more stable and stronger. It's useful to do so if you haven't squatted in years and are first getting into this training. This is called paradoxical breathing. It is recommended for use with weights as it creates a 'virtual belt' that helps to stabilize everything.

Of course, as soon as possible move into the anatomical style. This will also allow you to gain flexibility as you won't be tensed up from breathing in.

For more on the principles behind breathing, as well as tons of different breathwork, please see one of my most popular books, *Upgrade Your Breath*.

When you're working to improve your endurance, having a rhythmic breathing style is key. Breathing in and out in a relaxed manner, the same for each rep in the anatomical style, will allow you to go for long periods of time.

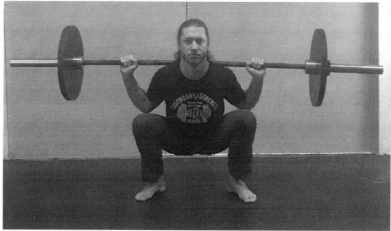

Typically, different breathing styles are used in barbell squats as compared to bodyweight squats

Key Points and Mistakes

There are a few common mistakes made in squatting. These can show imbalances in the body that may need correcting. They can also cause injuries if overdone so they're something to be watchful for.

Low Back Rounding

For most people when they reach the bottom position of a squat the lower spine will round. The tail bone tucks in.

There are some "spine experts" that say you should never do this. I believe the body can move in any way it can move and do so safely. With bodyweight squats this is especially not a problem. Under a heavy load like in barbell back squats, the exercise is typically limited to a parallel thigh level range of motion to prevent going into this low back rounding area. And that is fine for that exercise.

But don't think that it is dangerous to move beyond that when you're unloaded. It is okay for your lower back to round at the bottom position. As you improve your flexibility even more, you can keep your entire back straight too. The natural and most comfortable position for most will be with the lower back rounded. As with many things, there is no one right answer here, just different applications for each way of doing it.

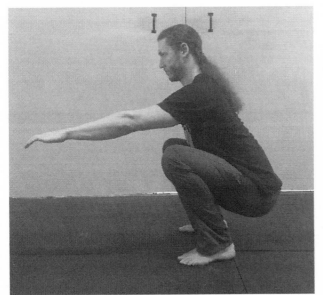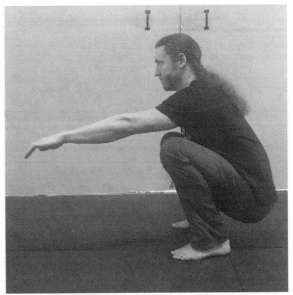

A normal more comfortable position with the lower back rounded I shown on the right, versus keeping as the whole back as straight as possible as shown on the left.

Knees Caving In

Knees caving in becomes more apparent under heavier loads or at the limits of your flexibility. The knees will cave inwards as you squat. The general rule of thumb you want to follow is to have your knees track over your toes the entire time you are in the squat. That means that the knee and the foot are pointed in the same direction throughout the movement.

A helpful cue is to force your knees slightly to the outside as you squat. If available, a partner can put their hands to the sides of your knees to help give this cue. Another option is to put bands around the legs near the knees to exert a constant pull that will force the hip abductors to work more.

Not Even Footed

This issue can lead to the previous one. While it's easier to see the movement in the knees the problem may be starting in the feet. Many people do not walk or stand with even pressure on all areas of the feet. They favor one side or another. If it's the insides of the feet this will likely lead to the caving in of the knees.

A helpful cue here is to make sure you're pressing down on the outsides of the feet. This will often automatically correct the knees.

Too much pressure can be put on the outsides of the feet though it is less common especially in squats. But if that's the case, the same correction works going the opposite way.

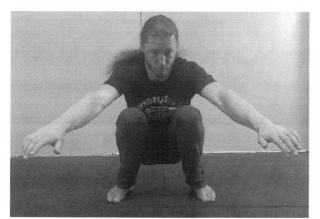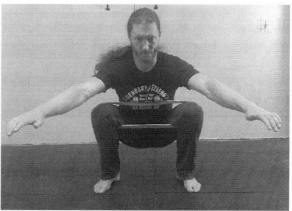

The first position commonly happens with squats, especially near a maximum strength level. One correction is shown in the second picture where bands are placed over the legs above the knees, so you must force your legs outward.

Sitting Back vs. Sitting Down

This cue can help some people to achieve a better squat. Instead of thinking of sitting down, sit back. That is reach your butt back as if you're sitting on a chair. (You'll naturally do this with the box squats because you must sit back.)

When you sit back your shins will stay mostly vertical. When you sit down your knees will come forward in front of your toes. Contrary to popular opinion, this is not a bad thing. Once again it is a natural movement of the body. With a heavy barbell on your shoulders you'll sit more back than down, but that's a function of the weight, and not so much because it will cause shearing forces on the knees. As long as the knees are tracking the toes, you should be fine sitting back or down.

Experiment for yourself. How does the squat feel differently when you sit back vs. when you sit down? Once again, neither of these is correct in all cases, just different uses for each.

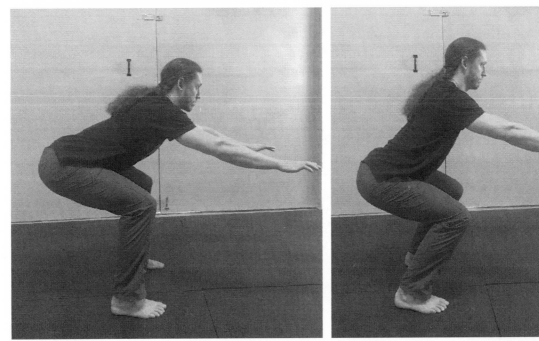

Pay attention to the shin position in both squats. This will be most clear around the parallel position as shown here because, when you reach rock bottom, you'll be in the same position with each. The left shows sitting back while the right shows sitting down.

Box Squats

The box squat is the ultimate way to both increase your flexibility over time and keep track of your progress. What you do is setup a box behind you as you stand in front of it ready to squat. Then squat back until you butt touches the box and stand up.

The box can be setup higher or lower to suit your level. Over time you continue to lower the height until you're squatting down "ass to grass".

I recommend working up to sets of 20 at each height.

So, what do you sit down onto? Personally, when it comes to bodyweight training, I have found that stackable aerobic platforms to be one of the best investments. These can be used for squats as well as much else. You can find a variety of options here:
https://legendarystrength.com/go/platform/

The reason that the stackable steps are useful is that usually you can get them in 4" increments like the set I have. Sometimes even smaller. Four-inch jumps works well enough with the basic squat.

And if you need smaller jumps you can put something like a book on top of the step to add another inch or two. In my gym I have a bunch of thin phonebooks for this purpose (as well as for phonebook tearing!).

Once again, these are not just useful for bodyweight squats. We'll be revisiting them again in the pistol squats and they're also useful for handstand pushups and pullups too.

Besides the steps, you can also use any sort of stable object. This includes chairs of different heights, stacks of wood, stairs, and much more. The important thing is to make sure that it is stable. Nothing is worse than hurting yourself because your platform fell over. If you're working with something like chairs it may be hard to find the progressive heights you need. But if you get creative you almost certainly can find at least a few options.

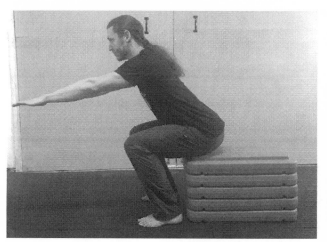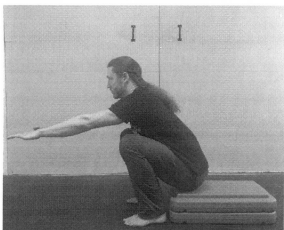

Doing box squats at different heights.

Different Box Squat Methods

There are three ways you can use the box.

1 - Touch and go. Once you've made contact reverse directions. This is the method described on the previous page.

2 - Sit down. Sit down completely on the box and allow yourself to relax, even if just for a split second. Then tighten up as needed and raise up.

3 - Rocking. Here you're using momentum to help you. Sit down fully but don't relax. Instead rock back, then forwards and use that momentum to help you come up.

Sitting down and relaxing is the hardest one because you must generate all the power and you eliminate the stretch reflex. That is because your muscles build elastic recoil as you control the negative.

Rocking is the easiest as you're adding momentum which will propel you upwards. And that means the touch and go method is in the middle. To sum up, in order of difficulty, easiest to hardest it goes:

1. Rocking method
2. Touch-and-go method
3. Sit down method

To keep things simple, you can just stick with the touch-and-go method. But if you want to mix it up then bring in all three variations. You'll want to work on different heights with them. For instance, you may be able to do rocking box squats at 20" and only do the sit down at 24". Ultimately, you want to work down to the lowest heights with the sit-down method.

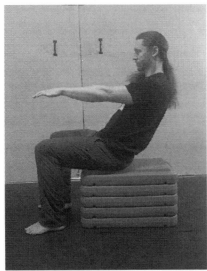 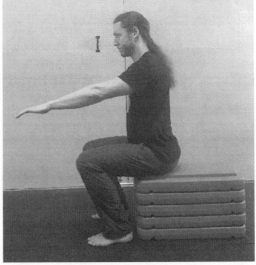

On the left is the rocking method. On the left is the sit-down method. Compare to the previous pictures where the touch-and-go method is used.

Prying the Hips

Here's another helpful way to improve your flexibility. Squat down as low as you can comfortably go, taking a wider stance than normal.

Shift your weight from side to side as you work to open up your hips more. You can raise on the toes or heel and move the feet side to side. Try bringing one leg closer or further out. The point is to move around to open up the space.

You can also take your elbows and push against the insides of your knees and thighs to "pry open" your hips. Use this in combination with moving around and you'll feel like you can create more space in the hips which will allow you to get a little lower.

This is especially useful when you can get into the bottom position but it's not quite comfortable yet. Still this can be used at any level. To be safe, you may want to have a wall or something nearby you can grab onto if you need help getting back out of this position.

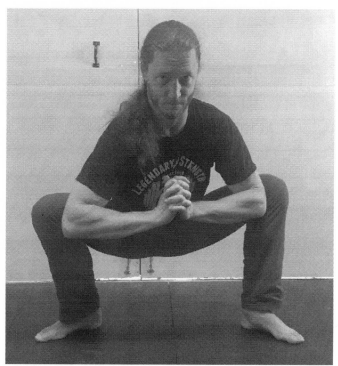

Notice the shifting of the weight as well as using the arms to pry open the hips.

Using a Support/Pulling Down

Also try grabbing onto the door handles of an open door, a cross bar on a power rack, or something similar, and squatting back. By having something to pull on you can often get even lower.

Secondly, instead of thinking of lowering to the ground, try thinking of pulling yourself down into position. This change of frames will give you a different feel on the exercise from a slightly different use or sequencing of the muscles.

If this is useful for improving your flexibility and squat than do it. If it's not for you, then don't.

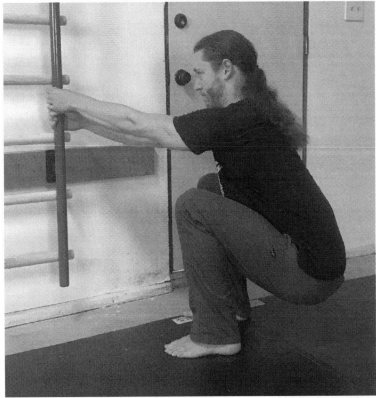

Holding onto a stable object allows you to sit further back.

Goblet Squat

The goblet squat is a weighted exercise, usually done with a kettlebell although a dumbbell works just fine. The reason I include it is that working with weight can help you increase your flexibility. The added weight assists you in getting into a lower position. (Of course, it will also require more strength to squat when supporting any weight but in this a relatively light weight is used.)

If you're working with a dumbbell you can grab both hands over the handle with the plates pointing upwards and downwards.

With a kettlebell you can hold it by the horns, that is the handle. The kettlebell can be facing down, the normal position, or you can flip it upwards so that it is bottoms up.

Feel free to use this exercise for strength, for flexibility and even to help you add reps. If you occasionally work with a light weight for high reps, when you go back to unweighted squats they'll feel even easier and you can do more of them.

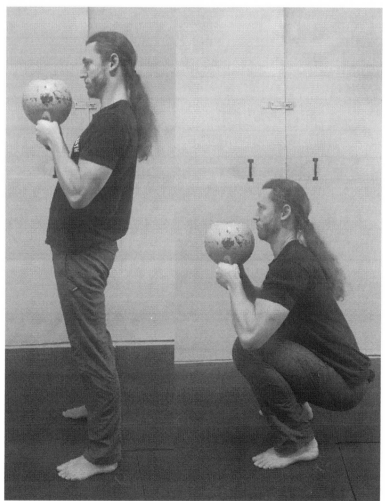

Great to make the exercise harder strength-wise and to help increase your flexibility.

Training for a Full Range of Motion

Besides working on the form, using various tricks to allow you to get down lower, your main plan of action will be the box squats. It is essential you set something up so that you can raise and lower the height, preferably by a couple inches at a time. The more incremental you make it the easier it will be.

Test yourself out to see what your maximum squatting depth is currently. I recommend that you write it down.

Increase the height a couple inches from that and that will be your starting height. Start with sets of 10 reps (if you must do less you certainly can).

In the beginning, you may only want to do 3 sets. Ease into this training slowly if you haven't done anything like it before, or at least not in a long time.

Our aim is daily training, so you don't want to do too much on the first day and leave yourself too sore to workout the next. Once you've gotten your baseline measurement and done your first workout the fun begins.

Everyday you're going to squat. Sometimes go with a higher height then normal. This will be easy for you. So, increase the volume you do. This can be more total sets. This can be more reps in each set. It can also be both.

Sometimes go with a medium to hard range of motion. You'll be doing less volume, but still work on increasing it from workout to workout.

Occasionally test yourself for a new depth and see how much you've improved. You can do a few single repetitions of this.

Why every day? Think of squatting as a skillset. By training often, the muscles of the legs will become conditioned to the strength and flexibility demands, more so than if you trained less often. Because we want to increase your squatting skill we do it every day. Later, when we up the volume or intensity, we can ease back in frequency, but for now every day is ideal.

You'll see in this training plan a few things. You're not just working on the flexibility though that is the main goal. By changing up the range of motion you'll be working the legs somewhat differently on different days. You're also increasing your strength and endurance as you work here. Here is an example of what this might look like:

Day 1
Max depth 20"
3 sets of 10 reps at 24"

Day 2
5 sets of 12 reps at 24"

Day 3
8 sets of 15 reps at 28"

Day 4
4 sets of 6 reps at 22"

Day 5
8 sets of 20 reps at 28"

Day 6
6 sets of 3 reps at 24"

Day 6
5 sets of 20 reps at 24"

Day 7
8 sets of 2 reps at 20"

Day 8
New max depth at 16"
3 sets of 6 reps at 20"

This is just an example. Your own training may take longer, or it could be faster progress as well. When doing this if you feel you need a day off to rest than take it. But simply by continuing this journey you will make it to rock bottom squats within some amount of time.

30 Minute Squat Challenge

The rock-bottom squat of which this module is focused is the first focus because it is a natural human movement. It's only with our over-use of chairs and lack of use of this position that most people in Westernized countries have lost this ability.

In other places where sitting at a desk, in a car, or in front of a TV for many hours each day doesn't take place, where chairs aren't as abundant, the full squat is used as a resting position. People play games in it. They relieve themselves by popping a squat, which happens to be better for elimination too than sitting on a toilet. For those still engaged in collecting their own food, a full squat is useful in both hunting and gathering.

The aim is not to power through the difficulty of getting yourself into position but learning to relax and be comfortable in it. It really is a resting position.

Once you can get into that bottom position, a challenge you can go after is to spend a total of thirty minutes each day in it. Credit goes to Ido Portal, a master of movement, for this idea. This will help transform the rock bottom position from something that might be a bit tough, into something that comes easily and naturally.

Take breaks at work and get in a squat. Converse with a friend from the squat position. I'm not going to recommend going to the bathroom in a hole in the ground outside, but I'm sure you can find other opportunities to hold that bottom position. (Instead I advocate a toilet, but also using a squatty potty.) Another good option since many of us spend time watching TV is to do it then.

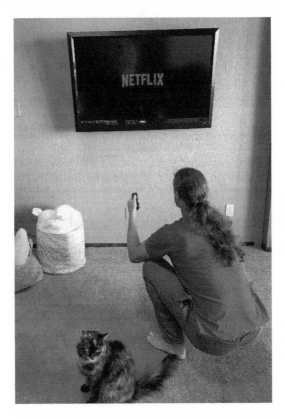

Do a minute here, two minutes there, until you've totaled 30 minutes for the day. Of course, work up to this amount if you need too. Just five minutes of squatting per day is a good start. Then ten minutes and so on.

Note that this is not to spend thirty minutes straight in a rock bottom squat. If you want to do that you can. I certainly have. But instead, the aim is to spread it throughout your day, which will bring about more benefit as it gets you using your natural human movement more often. You know, moving like a human is supposed to move.

Module 2 - Squat Variations

We've covered the basic squat and how to improve in it. Now it's time to move into variations of the squat. These change up how the muscles of the legs are used. Some may be easier, some harder. First off, we just work on changing position in how the feet and thus the legs are setup. This includes some lunge positions. And finally, we add resistance, make them explosive and do a few other things with the squat to make it harder.

Hindu Squat

This is one of the major variations to play with. Whereas the basic squat we covered has you squatting flat footed, the main difference here is that as you squat down you raise up onto the balls of your feet. This will target the quads and calves more than a flat-footed squat, while minimizing the work of the glutes.

In addition, this move is done with a cyclical breathing and rowing motion of the arms. At the top position you start with your arms straight out in front of you. Breathe in as you pull your arms to your chest. Raise up on your toes as you squat down and bring your hands to the floor. Explosively blow out the air at the bottom as you swing your arms up and come to standing. Repeat.

Strive to maintain a straight and upright back. It is natural to lean forward a little as you do this movement especially at speed, but the classic move has you having as upright a back as possible.

This move can be done for very high reps which will be talked about in the next module.

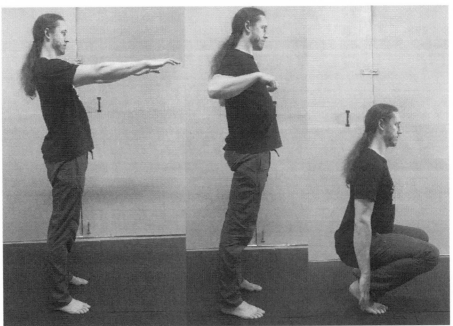

The Hindu squat is very rhythmic in nature. Great for high repetitions.

Close Legs/Feet Together Squat

This exercise increases the flexibility demands of the flat-footed squat. You can start with a closer than normal stance and over time keep moving the feet closer, until they are touching. By having your feet touching you must counterbalance your weight and be able to hold a flexible position at the bottom. For this reason, it is useful as a lead-up skill to the one-legged squat and will be discussed more later.

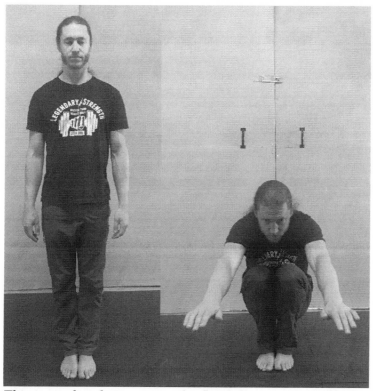

This immediately increases the flexibility required to squat.

Wide Squat

A wide squat will tend to work the hips and glutes more than other squats. As already discussed this can be useful in also increasing your hip flexibility.

One thing to remember is to keep your knees pointed over your toes. When your feet go wide it is more natural to turn them more outwards instead of having them point straight ahead. Thus, the knees should also be pointed more outward.

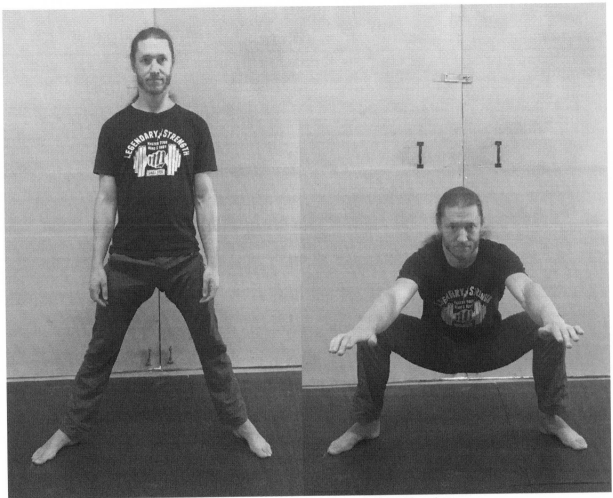

This wide position focuses on hip and glute development.

Sumo Squat

The Sumo Squat is built on top of the wide squat. Its name comes from the Sumo wrestlers who regularly practice it. As this exercise works more of one leg at a time it will require more strength.

After doing a wide squat pick one leg up into the air then bring it down (the stomp is optional) as you come into the next squat. Usually you switch sides from rep to rep although you could choose to focus on doing the same leg over and over.

An alternative version has you pick up the leg and then circle it around before coming down.

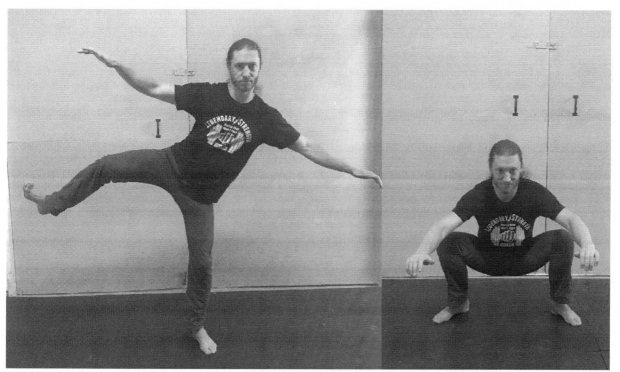

A variation of the wide squat that is more dynamic in nature.

Plie Squat

The Plie Squat comes from ballet. But don't make the mistake of thinking it's for sissies because it's one of the more difficult two-legged squat variations.

Here you're going to bring your heels together with the toes pointed outwards. Ideally you want them fully pointed to the sides, but this requires good flexibility to do. If you can only get part of the way that is fine for now.

As you descend in a squat you're going to raise up on the toes. Descend as deep as you can then come back up. This is an even better quad strength developer than Hindu squats. Typically, the arms come up and to the outside for balance.

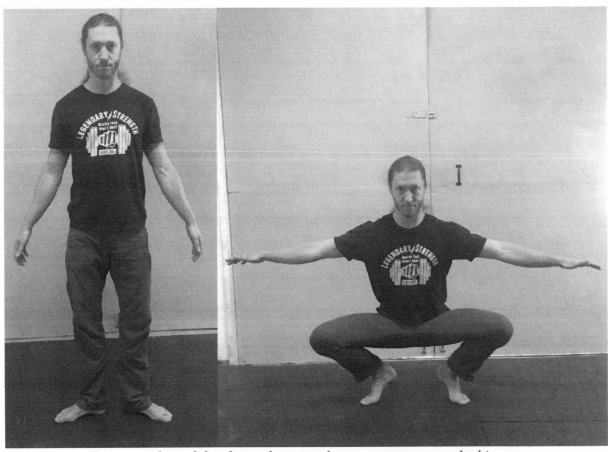

A phenomenal quad developer that can also serve to open up the hips more.

Circular Squats

In the circular squat you favor one leg as you come down and the other as you come up. Both legs will stay placed firmly on the ground you just shift your torso and hips over the main leg to be used. Thus, your body makes a circle as you squat. This is a helpful exercise to build strength for one-legged squats.

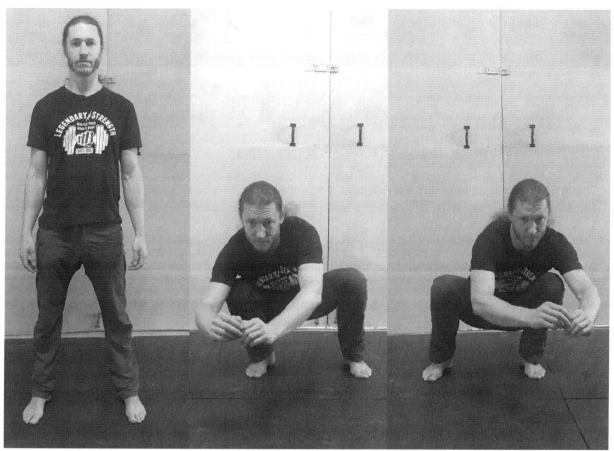

More emphasis is placed on one leg at a time in this squat variation.

Split Stance

Every squat we've done so far, even though foot position has changed, has remained in a neutral position, that is with the feet on the same plane. Here we're going to step one foot in front of the other, still about shoulder width apart.

As you squat down the front foot will stay flat footed as the back leg raises up on the toes. Make sure to work both sides, switching with foot is forward.

Try doing a bunch of squats with one stance, or alternating stance from rep to rep. You can play with wide or close stance variations with the split stance too.

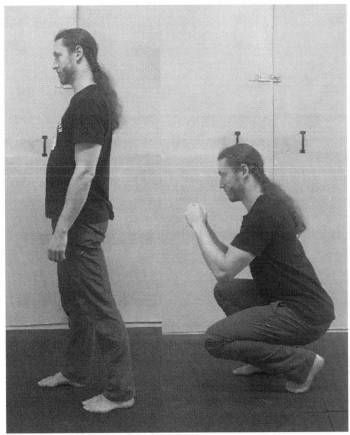

Half lunge and half squat. Simple yet very effective variation.

Lunges

The split stance squat is the start of a lunge, but with the lunge you are stepping into position. This exercise puts more emphasis on the working leg. Plus, there are many variations you can do based on the direction you step.

In a lunge you start in a normal standing position. Step one foot forward, with a larger than normal step. This forward foot will be flat footed. Bend the leg as the other foot stays in place but raises up onto the ball of the foot. Touch your knee to the ground (do not slam it). Press back up into your original standing position.

Variations include:

Alternating lunges – With each rep you step with the opposite foot.

Backwards lunges – Instead of stepping forward step backwards.

Walking lunges – Instead of pushing back to your original position push forward into the next lunge. Can also be done backwards.

Around the Clock lunges – Try stepping to any direction besides forwards and back. You can rotate most or some of your body into the lunge position. Just make sure the knees are tracking the toes.

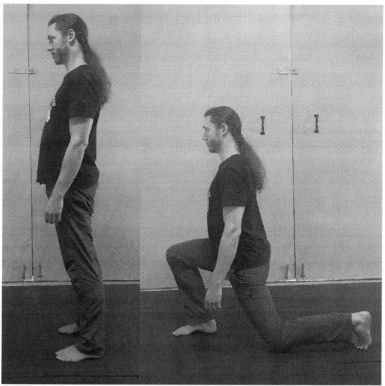

The brother of the squat that doesn't get nearly as much attention as it deserves.

Side to Side Squat/Cossack Squat

This is like a lunge but in a different position. Also great for flexibility.

Start in a wide squat. Descend to one leg while keeping the other straight. The foot you're squatting onto should remain flat on the floor. The other foot can be pointing up in the air.

You can raise up to standing as you do reps, or you can slide from side to side without coming up much. This exercise isn't often done with high reps but is more for stretching.

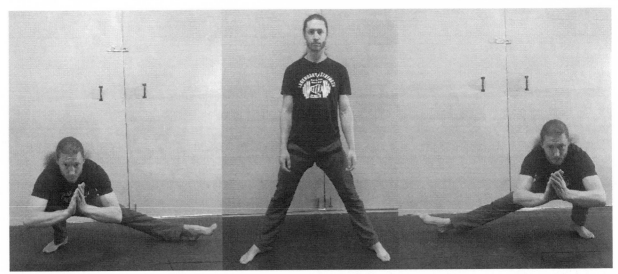

Great for increasing your flexibility even more.

Cross Leg Squat

Getting off the floor can take you through many squat and lunge positions. This is one way I like to get off the ground. If you're sitting with your legs crossed rock your weight forwards and, pressing on the sides of your feet, extend your legs until you come to a standing position.

You can also work cross leg squats without sitting on the ground. Don't do too many, but this can be a useful way to work your legs in an awkward position, with odd stress on your knees to strengthen your weak points.

It's interesting to note that this squat and sitting down and getting up off the floor in it, was shown in a study to be a good predictor of living in old aged people. That if you couldn't do it, you were more likely to die of all causes. More details can be found in The Stand-Up Challenge. https://legendarystrength.com/stand-up-challenge/

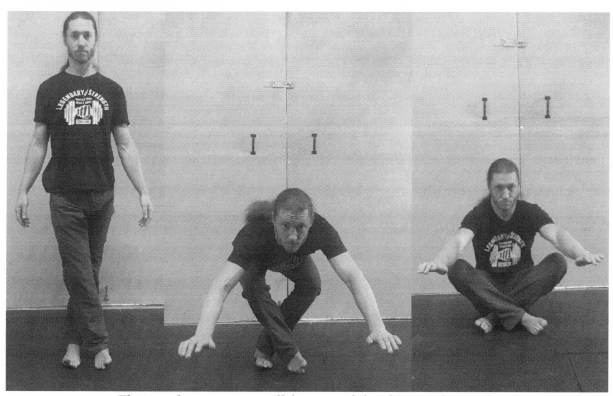

This is a fun way to get off the ground that few people can do.

Rollback Squat

Remember the rollback squat that was done as one of three methods with the box squat? If you're done with the boxes, the same move can be done on the ground to do a full rollback squat.

If you use a fair amount of momentum this can be easier than just the basic squat, especially if you have difficulties in holding that bottom position. But it can also be made harder by relying on less and less momentum. For most people, unless you can touch your butt to the ground in a squat, you'll still need some momentum to get back to your feet.

If you roll back all the way, to what is called the plow position in yoga, this can be a useful dynamic flexibility exercise. Learn to flow with the movement and you can have lots of fun doing this for reps.

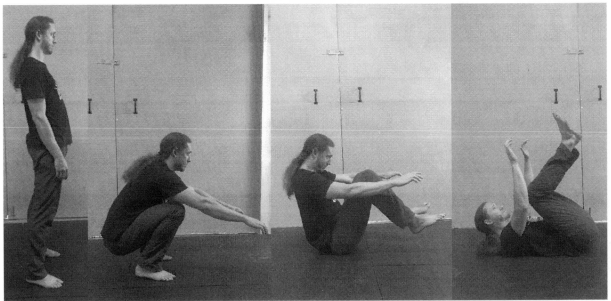

This move is easier than the basic squat when you use momentum, but it is also fun and can add flow to the movement.

Slow Squats

With any squat variation the default speed is at a regular pace. Not trying to move as fast as possible, but not going any slower than is needed either. By playing with the speed you can make any of the squat variations harder to do.

Try going up and down to a count of 10 or 30 and see how it is. Try doing ten of these in a row and you might be surprised and just how tough a couple reps can be.

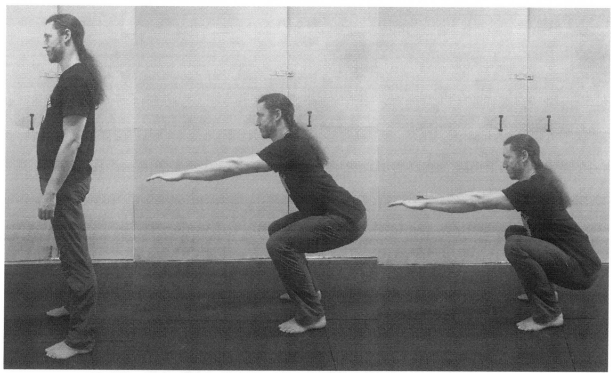

Try this with a 10 count up and a 10 count down and do that for reps.

Isometric Holds

Instead of always moving you can try holds in various parts of the squat. The horse stance is a classic from martial arts and something various people have held for very long times, even beyond an hour.

Another option is to isometrically press into the ground with your feet as you do these holds. This gives a different feel. Also try squeezing your feet together, without moving them, or spreading them apart. These additional isometric components can also be added to various moving squats.

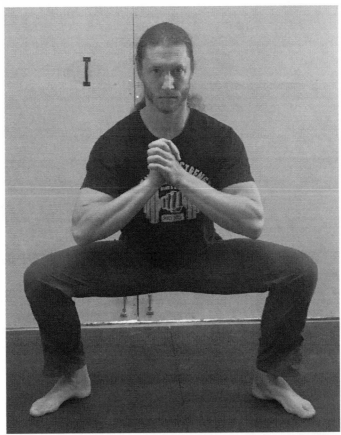

The classic horse stance can be held for long durations when trained.

Wall Chair

The wall chair is another form of isometric hold that works your legs in a semi-squat position. With your back against a wall, sit down, but with nothing under your rear. Your knees and hips should be at 90-degree angles. It is through pressing into the ground with your legs and your back into the wall that you hold this position.

A good challenge to work up to is holding a wall chair for ten minutes. The key is to learn to relax as much as possible while still maintaining the hold.

Variations include adding weight to the wall chair or doing a one-leg version.

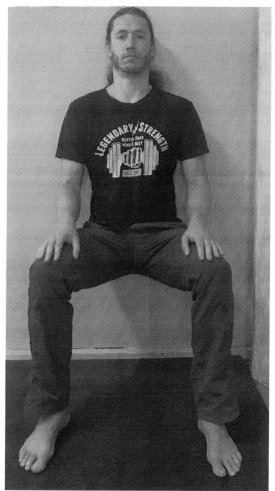

The wall chair is an isometric people love to hate.

Jumping Squats

Since handling your bodyweight soon becomes quite easy we need a few ways to make it more difficult. There are basically three options. Add resistance, go to one leg and add speed and explosiveness. All of them are good and this next series of movements covers the last option.

When you're jumping you normally don't descend into a full squat. You won't jump as high as if you only do a partial squat. But for the sake of this exercise to train the legs more explosively we will use a full squat.

Take a normal flat-footed squat position. Go into a full squat. From the bottom accelerate as fast as you can. You want to start jumping from the bottom and not only be explosive at the top.

You can work on doing the biggest jumps you can, or just get a moderate height and going for reps. You'll quickly find out how much tougher any jumping makes your cardiovascular system work.

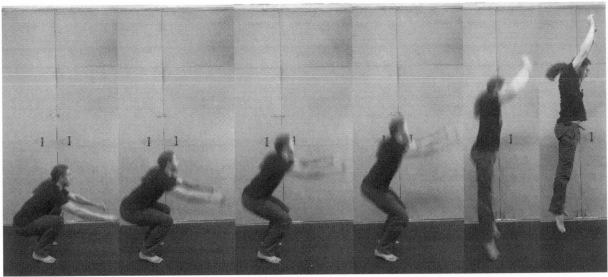

Make sure you have overhead space to jump as high as possible.

Squat Box Jump

Here we get a progressive component that can be used with jumping. You can setup boxes to any height. Just make sure they're a stable surface that can handle your weight.

There are two variations. You can do a full squat which will be harder, or just jump onto the box as you normally would.

For a normal jump here is the basic form. Squat slightly, no more than a quarter of the way as you aggressively push your hips back. Your arms will also swing down. Swing your arms forward as you snap the hips and jump off the ground.

For the full squat jump, it's the same as the jumping squat covered earlier, except now you land on the box.

To become even better at jumping work on how you land. Surprisingly enough, this will improve how far and high you can jump.

Or if you want less impact on your joints, don't jump down, but step down instead.

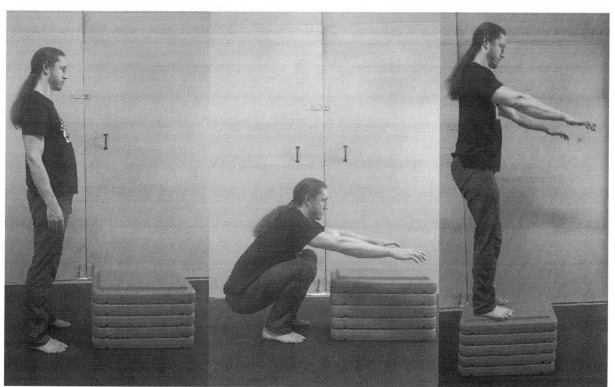

Try working all different heights.

Hindu Jumper Squat

The Hindu Jumper Squat is a bit more difficult than the regular Hindu Squat. Here when you explode upwards with your arms and legs you'll also jump forward about a foot. Then as you breathe in and row your arms back you jump back and descend into the squat. This requires a little more strength but is primarily for wind.

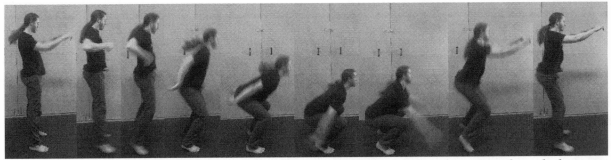

It may be hard to see the dynamic nature of this exercise in a picture but it's only a slight jump forwards and back with each rep.

Frog Jumps

Get into the bottom of a squat position. Staying in this position, jump up, without extending your hips. You can also travel forwards, to the sides and backwards.

Famous strongman George Jowett found this to be one of the best calf developers while jumping on the toes, which is another variation you can do.

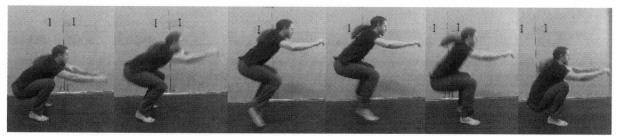

The flat-footed frog jump builds explosiveness in the bottom portion of a squat.

Jumping Lunge

Jumping from one lunge position to the next takes this exercise and makes it much tougher to do. Make it even harder by jumping high with each jump.

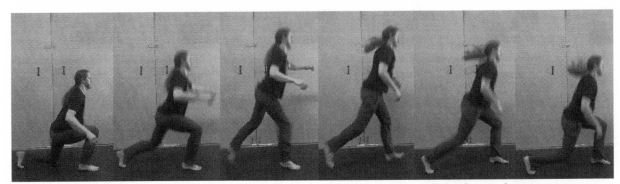

One of the best, yet simplest, cardio exercises you can do with bodyweight exercise.

Knee Jump Squat

Take a kneeling position on the ground. This is commonly called the seiza posture.

Snap the arms and the hip upwards, jumping, and come to the bottom of a squat. From here you can stand up then resume your position, kneel back down, or if you're on a padded surface you can also jump back down.

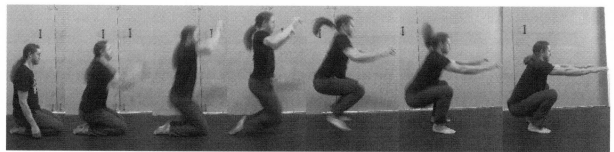

Not usually done for reps this quick exercise can get you off the ground fast.

Cable Squats

Adding resistance is another method of progression. Since the legs are strong this makes a barbell a great choice. You can also use kettlebells and dumbbells in a variety of ways, like in the goblet squat mentioned previously.

Another option to add resistance is to use cables or bands. Simply stand on the bands and loop the other end over your neck. The portable power jumper from Lifeline works great for this: http://www.legendarystrength.com/go/ppj/

This can be done with any version of the squat already covered, though some work better than others. With bands the more stretch that happens the harder it becomes so there will be more resistance at the top and less at the bottom.

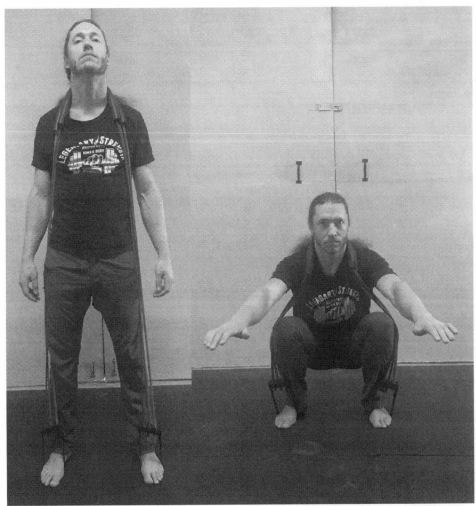

Cables are a great way to add resistance to make your legs work harder and they can still be done for high reps.

Weight Vest Squats

Another option to up the intensity while keeping it a bodyweight squat predominately is to put on a weight vest. This means you can add weight, but it still has the same exact feel as a bodyweight squat.

Of course, with a weight vest you can do any of the variations covered here.

I own, use and like the ZFOSports 80 lb. weight vest which is available at: https://legendarystrength.com/go/weightvest/

You can increase or decrease the weight in 4 lb. increments meaning you can make small adjustments over time. There are other weight vests available too. I've heard good things about Mir weight vests but have not personally used them.

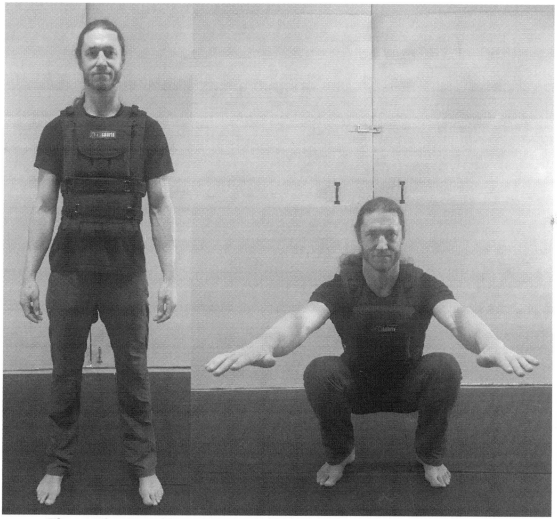

The weight vest adds resistance while still feeling like a bodyweight squat.

Training for 100 Squats in One Set

A great benchmark to go for is to do 100 bodyweight squats in a single set. This requires both leg strength and endurance. You might be amazed to know there's many otherwise strong and muscular people that would fail at this test, due to their lack on conditioning. Building up to 100 reps straight can be as simple as adding more volume over time in a few different ways.

The following workout plan is best done three times a week. Let's say you start off and the best you can do in a single set is 30 reps. For this training plan, you're going to work squats three times a week. Try to do each set with about 2 minutes of rest between them.

Workout 1
3 sets of 20

Workout 2
4 sets of 20

Workout 3
5 sets of 20

Workout 4
3 sets of 25

Workout 5
4 sets of 25

Workout 6
5 sets of 25

Workout 7
3 sets of 30

Workout 8
4 sets of 30

Workout 9
5 sets of 30
…

I think you get the point so far. This double system of progression has you increasing sets and then reps a little at a time from workout to workout. You could continue like this as long as you don't plateau.

Once you build up to sets of 50 in these workouts I think you'd find that you're ready for the challenge. Take an extra day or two off for more rest. Then with a little mental toughness push yourself for a new max. If you make it congratulations. If not, just continue working a little more and you'll get there soon enough. There are more tips on going to even higher numbers in the next module.

In the beginning you'll want to do this with just the basic squat, but then…

Training Program for a Variety of Squat Forms

We can take the exact same plan and start mixing in all the different variations. Because these variations are harder, each workout will be tougher than just sticking to the basic squat. Once again, you can do these three times a week. And, if you've been working the previous plans, you could also likely do it four times a week too.

Workout 1 – Hindu, Circular and Jumping Squats
3 sets of 20

Workout 2 – Hindu Jumper, Close Squats and Split Stance (both left foot forward and right foot forward in two different sets)
4 sets of 20

Workout 3 – Sumo, Cossack, Lunge (Left and Right), Squat Box Jump and Rollback
5 sets of 20

Workout 4 – Repeat versions from workout 1
3 sets of 25

Workout 5 – Repeat versions from workout 2
4 sets of 25

Workout 6 – Repeat versions from workout 3
5 sets of 25

Workout 7 – Repeat versions from workout 1
3 sets of 30

Workout 8 – Repeat versions from workout 2
4 sets of 30

Workout 9 – Repeat versions from workout 3
5 sets of 30
…

As before, keep on repeating as you increase the amount of reps you do in each set. As its written, you repeat the same variations after three workouts, but you could just as easily mix it up each time. You could even pick random variations every time you train.

Alternating Long and Short Set Workouts with Variety of Squats

If you want to work a bit harder but less often, here is a good plan for training just twice a week. Here you will be doing one max set in one workout, trying to push upwards the number you can handle. The other workout is done with shorter sets, but more overall volume.

These are just example variations and numbers:

Workout 1 – Hindu Squats
One set of 100

Workout 2 – Close, Wide, Lunges (Left and Right), Cossack, Jumping, Weight Vest, Rollback, Circular, Knee Jump
10 sets of 20

Workout 3 – Basic Squats
One set of 125

Workout 4 – Repeat versions for Workout 2, plus Split Stance (Left and Right)
12 sets of 20

Workout 5 – Hindu Squats
One set of 150

Workout 6 - Repeat versions for Workout 4, plus Slow Squats and Frog Jumps
14 sets of 20

Workout 7 – Basic Squats
One set of 175

Workout 8 – Repeat versions for Workout 2
10 sets of 25

Workout 9 – Hindu Squats
One set of 200

Workout 10 – Repeat versions for Workout 4
12 sets of 25
…

And so on.

Module 3 – Training for Hundreds or Thousands of Reps Straight

This is the shortest module of the bunch as we don't introduce any new exercises. Instead it's all about taking what you've already learned and advancing it further.

I first got into serious bodyweight training from Matt Furey, one of the biggest proponents of the Hindu squat. He set a benchmark for people to achieve 500 of these squats within 15 minutes. Working the training plans from the previous module will get you there. And I have a few more tips especially as you get to the higher rep counts.

I encourage you to not just work with one variation of the squat. Work with several variations and you'll have greater well-rounded development. For instance, the Hindu squats work the quads more, whereas wide squats will develop your hips. But if you're doing lots of reps of all different kinds it will add up to you being able to do a lot in one set and style when you choose to go for it.

When it comes to bodyweight squats once you get to a certain level of strength and endurance you can always do one more. It's more a matter of mental toughness than strength or endurance once you're here. Your muscles may burn, and you may be very sore the next day, but you can choose to keep going. Here the difficulty of one rep is less than is basically recovered in the time to do it, thus you can keep going.

In fact, there's a good chance that this is true right now for you…you just might not know it!

One day when I was hanging out with my friends we were talking about reaching 500 Hindu squats. My friend said that he could do that. Another friend of mine and I called B.S. on him. He was adamant, so a bet was put in place. He started cranking out the squats, one after the other. 200…300…he was hurting, he was struggling, but he kept going. Soon enough he was at 400 and then he hit the goal of 500. He won the bet and I have to say it was worth it to watch that happened as it expanded my mind.

In my very next workout, I easily hit some new records for myself. I didn't go straight to 500, but I knew I could go further. I knew I could do that if I wanted to. It was like a switch got flipped in my mind.

Now this does come with a warning. My friend was sore for about a week straight. You know that kind of soreness where you can't even walk straight? So, this does come with a caveat, but know that if you can do 100 bodyweight squats, you can pretty much keep going if you're willing to tap into your mental toughness.

A goal of 500 can be fun to shoot for but it's not necessary. Once you can do 200 straight I would work on building the intensity of the movement, which is what the next chapter is all about. Although these high reps are a great starting point, like I said your endurance, and especially strength, gets to a point where you need more of a challenge, and endless reps isn't the most useful. Beyond this point you won't see increases in your strength and performance, at least I didn't. Some may disagree with me, but that is my own experience.

Here is what noted strongman and author Earle E. Liederman said on the subject in his book *Endurance,* "Without a definite objective I am sure that between one hundred and two hundred deep knee bends would give you sufficient endurance in the muscles of your thighs for all ordinary demands of daily life or emergencies."

Still for those that want to go further I want to give you additional tips and methods to get there.

My best ever single set of bodyweight squats was 1000 reps straight on Hindu squats. I did this as part of what I called the Ultimate Royal Court Challenge. The Royal Court was the main three exercises taught by Matt Furey. In addition to the Hindu squat, this included Hindu Pushups and the wrestler's bridge. In my challenge this was a 10-minute wrestlers bridge hold without using the hands and 250 Hindu pushups. The squats were done after those two all back to back!

I was doing this challenge as preparation for Matt Furey's Combat Conditioning Athlete of the Year, which I did win that year. It was this overpreparation that allowed me to win.

In training for this challenge, I never did more than 500 Hindu Squats at one time. But I did do two things that really helped. These will apply equally as well for working up to 100 reps in a single set or to 1000, or even beyond. Similarly, this could be done to build up to higher rep sets such as 100 reps of much more difficulty versions like the jumping squats too.

Spreading Squats Throughout Your Day

One method that will help you to extend your single rep sets is to do lots of volume. And one way to do lots of volume is not to do just a single workout session, but instead do those sets throughout the day. Pavel Tsatsouline talks about this as "greasing the groove." While his focus is usually strength and skill work, it can also work for endurance.

Try doing sets of 100 (or 20, 50 or 65, etc. depending on your level) throughout the day. Any one set won't be that hard but together you're building up to lots of volume. I recommend different variations for the sets but one third or half of them should be the kind you're shooting for in your one long set.

Since these are endurance sets you'll be getting winded and fatigued to some degree, but the point is to minimize that. In other words, if you max set is 100 don't try doing sets of 100. Instead do sets of 50 or so. Ultimately, you want all these sets to be relatively easy for you.

How many sets do you do? Aim for double the volume you want in a single set. So, for my goal of 1000 reps in a set, I would work up to 20 sets of 100 throughout the day. If your aim is 500 in a single set, you'd work up to 10 sets of 100, or 20 sets of 50. Keep in mind I said work up to. This means you may start with five sets, then the next day you're doing this you do six or seven sets, and so on.

You can do more total volume by spreading the work throughout the day, then you could in a single workout. This is because you have ample rest time. But be wary that more total volume likely leads to more soreness and necessary recovery time. This kind of training is best done maybe twice a week. And the frequency of training brings me to my next method...

Upping the Frequency

I was using the above method to help build my base. Once I had done 2000 total squats in a day, I switched gears.

I had never done more than 500 squats in a single set. I knew that it was all about mental toughness at that point. If I could do 500 well, then I could do 1000, even after the bridging and Hindu pushups too (which work the legs as well).

My next plan was to do a set of 500 but do it more frequently. I went through a week straight doing 500 Hindu squats every single day. The first couple days I was sore afterward but by the end I wasn't sore at all from this workload.

I conditioned my legs to not only withstand the work but be able to do so without impacting my ability the next day. Earlier in the section on progression I mentioned that frequency of training was a lesser factor of progression. But at certain times, like this one, it can be very effective.

And I wasn't just doing the squats either during this week. I was doing a 5-minute bridge and 100 Hindu pushups too. I mixed up the order that I did these different exercises from one day to the next.

Not only was I able to do this, but I got faster. The standard was to do that set of 500 Hindu squats in 15 minutes. Somewhere near the end of this week I was cranking them out in close to twelve minutes. The full workouts were taking somewhere between 20 to 25 minutes.

After that week I took a few days off to allow the recovery from what was certainly overtraining to take place. Then I went for the Ultimate Royal Court Challenge.

When I went for 1000 squat reps it was just a matter of keeping it up. The endurance was there, it was just mental toughness. In this case it did take over 30 minutes to do the squats. If I remember correctly it was somewhere around 32 minutes. Slower than I wanted to go but that was because of fatigue from the bridge and pushups before it. As a side note the squats were not the hardest part of this challenge, but instead the pushups.

Again, this is an example that can be adjusted to your level. Perhaps you can try sets of 125 each day and then set a new record for yourself of 250 after you take a day or two off.

Module 4 – Achieving the Pistol Squat

When it comes to bodyweight exercises the most natural form of upping the intensity of progression is to move onto one limb. When it comes to the lower body this is much easier than the upper body. Still this move can elude people. Thus, this section is all about what you can do to work up to it, and the following section is to take your mastery further. We'll start with the full movement then go back to regressed variations from there.

It's important to note that everything previous in this book will serve as the building blocks to get to this area. I would recommend you can do at least 100 straight reps of a few different forms of bodyweight squats. Specifically working on circular squats, split stance squats, and lunges will help as in all of those you work one leg more than another. The most important of squats already covered is the close leg squat. That will be talked about even more here.

Pistol Squats

Stand up tall. The leg you're going to be squatting on should be centered under your body, rather than shoulder width as that would cause you to fall. This means you're shifting the working legs hip slightly to the outside. The foot is pointed straight ahead.

Raise the other leg up in the air. Extend both arms forwards to act as a counterbalance. Squat down on your leg until your hamstring touches your calf then come back up.

When you're starting out with this move it will be tough, so you'll want to breathe in at the top or on the way down. You can use your breath to tighten up and then exhale forcefully to come out of the bottom. With practice you can switch to anatomical breathing as you go up in repetitions.

If you're doing reps of the one-legged squat the other leg should not touch the ground. In your training you may come up crooked every once in a while and need to touch your toe down to regain your balance. Or hop around on the one foot until you catch your balance. This is fine. But if you're going for an all-out set the general rule is that nothing can touch the ground besides the foot that is firmly planted on it.

What to do with the Free Leg?

There are three options for what you do with the free leg, shown in the order of difficulty:

1. Holding it with your hand
2. Keeping it relaxed
3. Keeping it straight

Holding the Free Leg

The first option is to hold onto your free foot with your hand. Usually it is by the same side arm, but you can cross over the body or use both hands too. This changes the feel of the exercise. By using your arm, you don't have to work at all to keep your leg up. It also keeps your torso far forward which can help in getting the balance. Lastly, it seems to bring together the whole movement as you're touching two different limbs together.

This can be a helpful version to do when first working on the movement. By holding onto your foot you're leaning for forward which counterbalances your weight. When the bottom position is tough to do, this version may help you to get it.

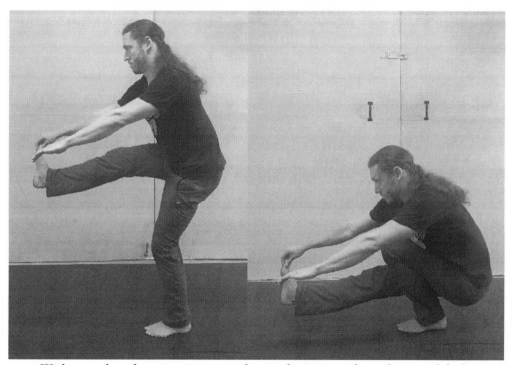

With your hand supporting your leg it changes up how the pistol feels.

Keeping the Free Leg Relaxed

For the most part when training pistols I keep my free leg relaxed. To me, this is the default style. You'll still have to hold it up off the ground, and at the bottom range of motion it will be mostly straight, but by keeping it as relaxed as you can you'll be able to do more reps with the working leg.

In doing this you don't want the foot to hit the ground unless that is your intention. You can use this free leg as a spot when you're starting out. The slight help in balance or pushing off can be a difference maker for you.

In this form you basically just want to keep the free leg out of the way.

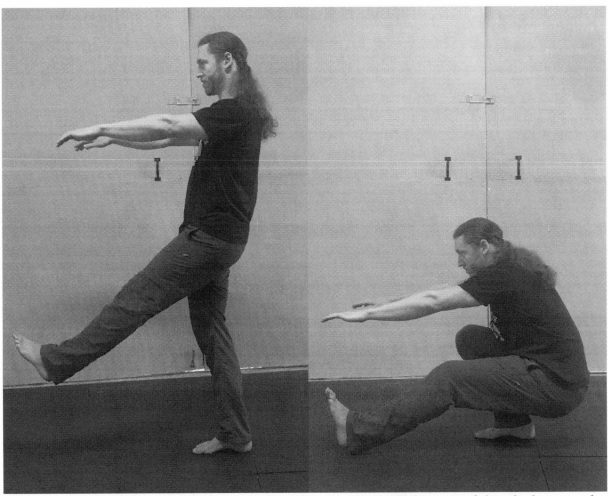

Here the free leg is kept as relaxed as possible. The leg stays off the ground, but the knee can be bent, and the hip is engaged as much as it needs to be, but no more.

Keeping the Free Leg Straight

The most difficult position is to keep it straight throughout the movement. This requires active flexibility on the part of the hip flexor to raise it up and for that reason, strength is required as well. It also looks better.

But in my opinion, it is not the focus of the exercise and can detract from it, which I why I mainly go with the relaxed option. If you're looking to work this free leg even more then go for it. This can be useful for martial artists or other people where dynamic flexibility is required.

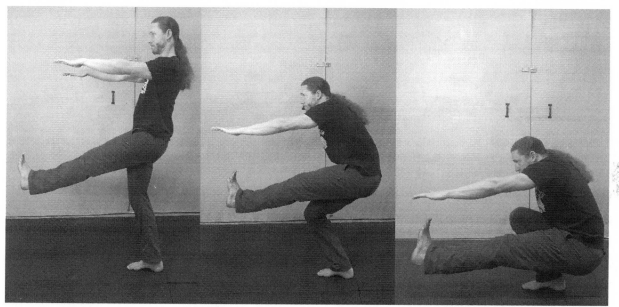

Notice that the free leg stays in the same parallel to the ground position for the entire movement which requires more strength and dynamic flexibility.

Flexibility and Close Leg Squats

For many people the problem in doing pistols is flexibility and not strength. As always there are ways to build up to what you need. The close leg squat is one of the best intermediate steps. At the bottom you'll notice your body is in the same position whether on two legs or one here. Besides a tiny shift to the side to get your weight more centered you'll have the same forward lean.

Something that can be stopping many people is a lack of dorsiflexion, that is the ankle being able to bend so that the foot and shin come towards each other. I've seen people lose this ability in always being taught to sit back instead of down. If you need to, go back to the earlier section where this was discussed and play with these squats again. Striving for a vertical shin position will make the pistol impossible to do as your knee must come over the toes to have your center of gravity over the foot and not be falling.

Use the close leg squat to develop this. Don't just do reps but get comfortable in the sitting position. (You could try a 30-minute challenge in the close squat!)

Also, the close leg squat is not just one move. You can inch your feet inward. Start with your normal squat stand and shift your feet in an inch at a time. You can work any step between this up until the feet are side by side touching.

As far as flexibility is concerned many big guys won't be able to do the pistol because their body mass will get in the way of them being capable of achieving the position needed to hold the bottom. If the free pistol is your goal you may have to lose weight, even muscle to do it.

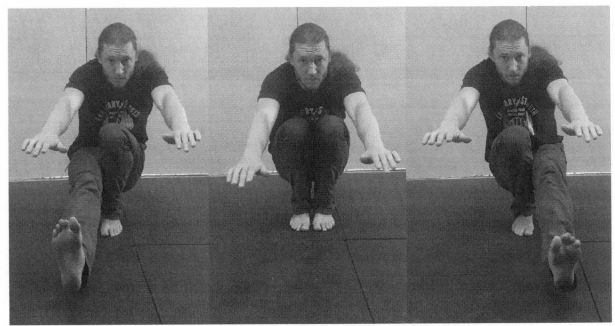

The weight shifts to the side slightly as the leg is raised.
Besides the counterbalancing lean to the side, the leg position is the same.

Counter Balance

Here is an exercise where adding weight can make it easier. If you take a small weight and hold it in front of you, this changes your center of gravity and can allow you to be sitting back more and get into the bottom position. The same concept as was covered in the goblet squat.

In a free pistol your weight must be balanced over the foot with a good portion towards the ball of the foot. With a counterbalancing weight your weight can be on the heel and your body will not need to flex forward as much.

In training the pistol, using a counterweight is fine. One method of progression is reducing the amount of weight you use. For instance, go from a 16kg kettlebell to 12kg, 8kg, then a 10 lb. plate, 5 lbs., 2 ½ lbs. You can use this is a form of progression to get to the free pistol, though it is not my favorite for this exercise.

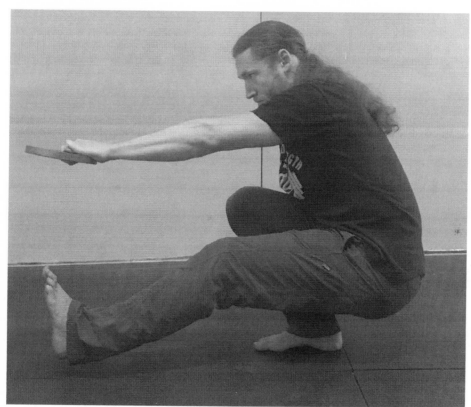

Holding a 5 lb. plate, because of leverage, makes the pistol easier.

Raised Heel

A way you can build up to pistols is to raise your heels up slightly. This can be in a shoe with a heel (please no high heels) or by sliding a weight plate under your heel. It allows you to do the move without the required dorsiflexion. I'd rather you progress with other methods then sticking with this one, as it reinforces bad habits. Still, I mention it as some people may find it useful.

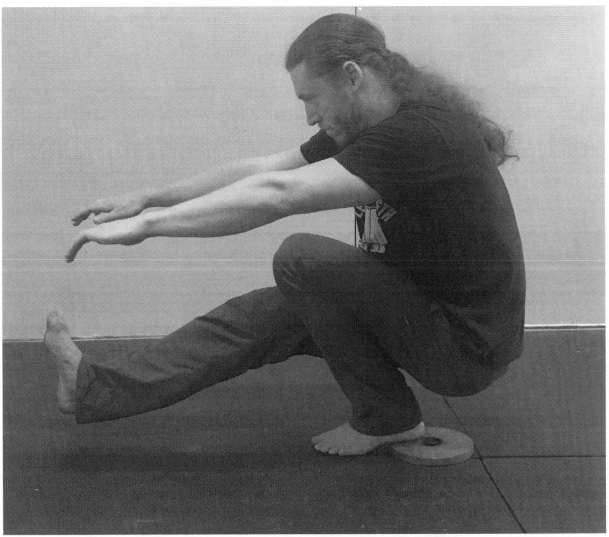

My heel is raised up with a 5 lb. weight plate under it.

Holding Onto Something

As in the two footed squats, you can hold onto a door knob, a power rack, or something else, as you learn the pistol. This will achieve the same effect as the counterweight, with you using as much force as needed to help you complete the move. I prefer the weight, as it moves more with you, but this is another option.

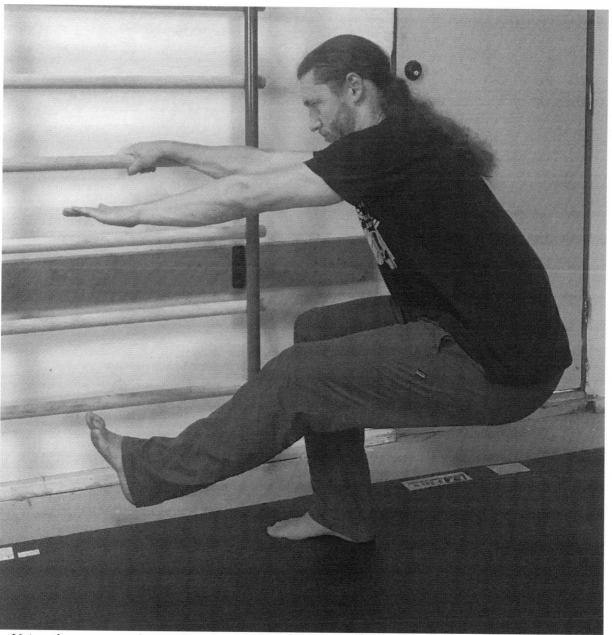

Using the power rack or a door knob allows you to sit more back and keep the weight on your heels making the pistol easier.

Gripping and Breathing Tip

This little tip I picked up from Pavel Tsatsouline at a Naked Warrior Seminar many years ago. Pavel is a big fan of keeping as tense as possible and adding tension where and whenever possible. One way of doing that is to tighten up parts of the body that aren't even involved in the exercise you're doing.

For the pistol that can be the hands. Descend into the pistol like you normally do. When you get to the bottom turn your open hands into tight fists as you exhale and explode upwards. You'll likely find that you moved faster and possibly even smoother than if you weren't to do this.

I don't recommend doing this all the time, but it's a useful trick to have when you're working near your limits. This is also useful to add to jumping pistols as covered in the next module as it helps you explode out of the hole.

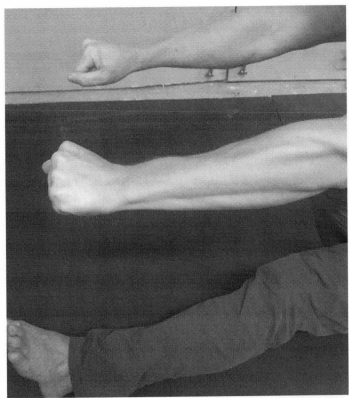

Explosively squeezing your fists out of the hole, aka the bottom of the pistol, can help generate strength to come up. This is especially useful with weights or explosive versions, but is also useful when you're starting out to reach your first reps.

Box Pistols

Our old friend the box is coming back. Just as this was the mainstay method of building up to a full range of motion in the squats, it will be used here for the same except you'll be on one leg. Setup the box in a stable manner and work to see how low you can go, touching your butt to it, then coming back up. As a reminder, there are three ways you can use the box, in order of difficulty:

1 - Rocking
2 - Touch and go
3 - Sit down

As with the earlier box squats with two legs, you can choose to just stick with the touch and go method or work with all three methods as you progress. Work on different heights with them. For instance, you may be able to do rocking box pistols at 20" and only do the sit down at 24". Smaller increments will make this even more progressive.

This is the best method to master the pistol squat. This is how I first achieved it with a couple months' worth of practice many years ago. Just take it a piece at a time. Increase your range of motion when you can and eventually you can do away with the boxes completely.

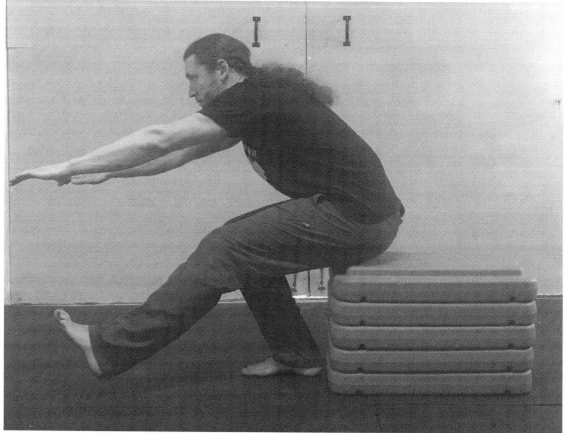

An example of the touch and go pistol at a limited range with the boxes.

Elevated One Legged Squat

Here is another method that you can use with boxes. Here you'll stand on top of them and squat down. The free leg no longer needs to be held in front of the body because you have height.

This was a favorite of Paul Anderson because he was too massive to do the classic pistol. In this way you can work unilateral strength in the legs without much demands on your flexibility.

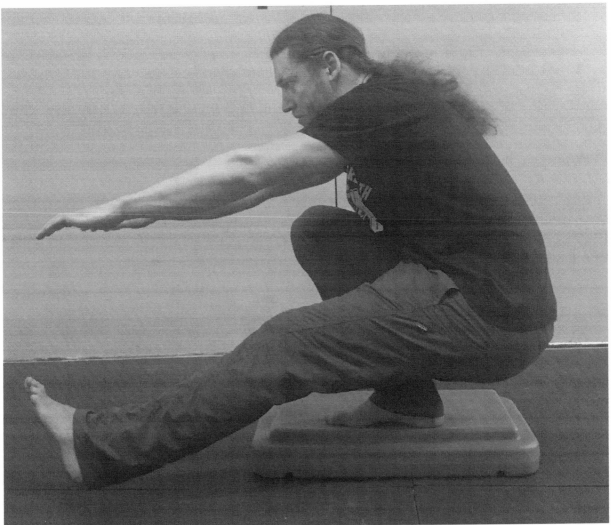

Not having to raise the free leg much makes this exercise easier on your flexibility.

Rolling Pistols

In the rolling pistol you do just like the rocking box pistols before, except that now you do it on the ground. The momentum makes this a little easier if you go with a little speed.

But it also requires a little more flexibility if you slow down the movement as you must squat all the way down, then reach to sit on the ground. And if you slow the momentum coming back to your foot can be tough to do. This culminates in the sit to pistol covered in the next module.

One tip is that when you're coming up get the foot as close to your butt as you possibly can. Then shoot your hands forward as if reaching so that you can get your weight over onto the foot.

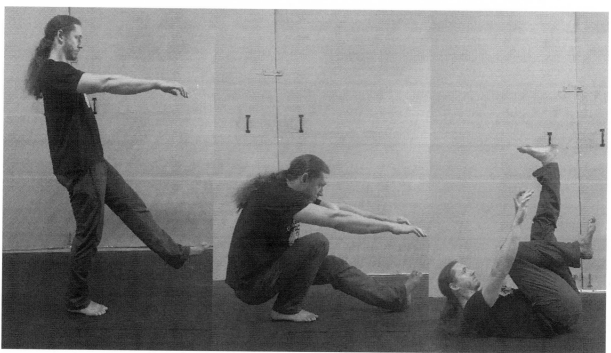

The rocking position on the ground.

Training to Achieve Your First Pistols

Just like the two-legged basic squat, we'll rely on the box pistol as the main method of training. Personally, this is how I achieved my first pistols after just a couple of weeks of training when following Pavel Tsatsouline's *The Naked Warrior*. https://amzn.to/2KYOtl4

Everything that was discussed before regarding box squats and training with them applies here. For that reason, I'm presenting the exact same workout plan except now that you work it with pistols on each leg instead of the basic squat. What this means is that the same progression will work just like before.

The only thing I've added is a single set of 20 close squats. This serves as a warmup and can be done incrementally so that your feet move ever closer until they are touching. Start with whatever width you need to go rock bottom then progress from there.

Once again, this training is best done daily in the beginning. After we've achieved the pistol and start adding significant volume, weight, explosiveness or other methods, then the frequency will be changed. Here is an example of what this might look like:

Day 1
Close Squats x 20
Max depth 20"
3 sets of 10 reps each leg at 24"

Day 2
Close Squats x 20
5 sets of 12 reps each leg at 24"

Day 3
Close Squats x 20
8 sets of 15 reps each leg at 28"

Day 4
Close Squats x 20
4 sets of 6 reps each leg at 22"

Day 5
Close Squats x 20
8 sets of 20 reps each leg at 28"

Day 6
Close Squats x 20
6 sets of 3 reps each leg at 24"

Day 6
Close Squats x 20

5 sets of 20 reps each leg at 24"

Day 7
Close Squats x 20
8 sets of 2 reps each leg at 20"

Day 8
Close Squats x 20
New max depth at 16"
3 sets of 6 reps each leg at 20"

This is just an example. Your own training may take longer, or it could be faster progress as well. When doing this if you feel you need a day off to rest than take it. Six days a week with one rest day works quite well.

Note that these workouts assume you're able to do the same amount with each leg, when there's a good chance that will not be the case. While striving for some amount of symmetry is good, it's okay for things not to be equal. After all, are you completely ambidextrous? No? Then I wouldn't expect your strength or flexibility to be either.

In this case, your right leg may be working at 20" while your left leg is lagging back at 24". As long as you're progressing forward with both you'll eventually get full pistols with each leg.

You may be able to just stick with the touch-and-go method, or if desired add in the rocking and sit-down methods too. Once you're low enough and do away with the box the rocking pistol becomes the rolling pistol, which is a good preliminary step right before the full bodyweight pistol.

Module 5 – Mastering the Pistol Squat

This chapter will cover a few different pathways to master the pistol. We'll discuss adding reps, adding weight, and other advanced variations.

Here are two benchmarks to aim for. Obviously, hitting your first free pistol is a huge goal. From there a good intermediate goal is 10 reps on each leg. Then shoot to achieve 20 reps on each leg.

Remember that these must be done without touching the other foot to the ground at all. When you've reached this goal, you've turned something that for many is a test of strength into the beginnings of one for endurance. You can choose to go even higher rep than this if you want, but once you're at twenty reps, I think aiming for added difficulty is the way to go.

If you want to go very high rep, then all the previously covered material applies the same here too.

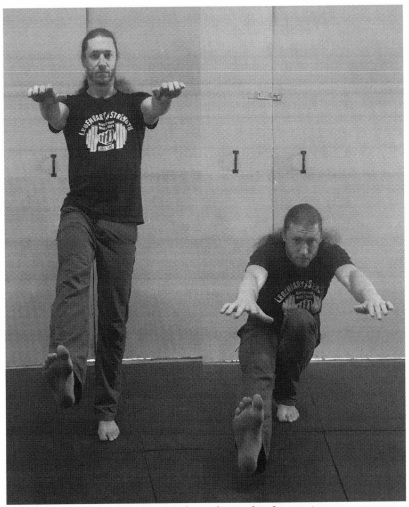

A regular pistol done from the front view.

Switching Legs

A way to get in lots of reps without over working the legs one at a time, is to do alternating pistols. Instead of doing as many reps as you can on a single leg at a time, switch legs every rep. You'll be able to do a lot more in this manner. Just switch legs at the top position.

Or you can also switch legs at the bottom position. Squat down on one leg. Bring your free leg in so you end in a close stance squat. Then raise up on the opposite leg from the one you just came down on.

Thus, you have two different options for the switch leg pistols.

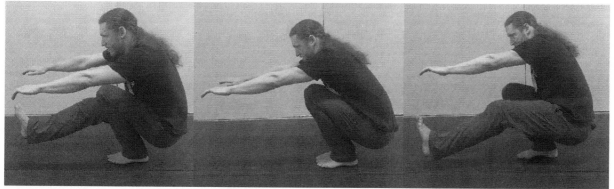

Switching legs while in the bottom position moves you through a feet-together squat.

Sit to Pistol

Just because you've acquired the flexibility and mobility to achieve the pistol, doesn't mean it ends there. In this move you go from a sitting position and, without momentum, shift up into the bottom of the pistol and then stand up. It's like the rollback pistol, but without any rolling or momentum used.

To do this you'll want to tuck your squatting leg in as close to your butt as comfortably possible. Your free leg will be straight out and resting on the ground. Reach your hands, and in fact your whole torso as far forward as possible. Press into the ground with your foot and shift your whole weight off the ground, raising the free leg too.

I find this to be a great warmup drill for more advanced one-legged squat work.

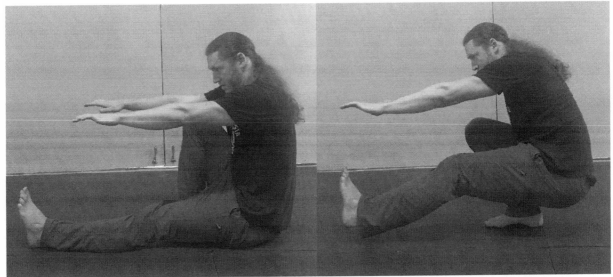

Reach far forward with your foot, hands and torso to move from sitting into a pistol.

Cossack Dance

Hold the bottom of a pistol then do a small aggressive jump and switch to the other leg. Much more explosive then the switching of legs done earlier. Requires a good command of the bottom position to be able to do it fast and go back and forth.

This can also be done on the toes to be in the more classic Russian style.

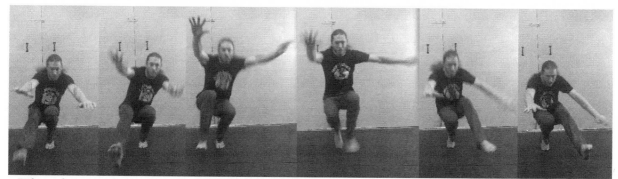

When doing a dynamic exercise like this one you may end up off balance to the sides like in the last picture. This is great training for not always being in a perfect position.

Jumping Pistols

By adding the explosive component to it you can further develop your strength. As discussed in earlier jumping squats, you're going to descend fully into the squat and then explode out as much as you can from the bottom position and not just jump with the last portion of the movement. Jump up and land in the same spot ready to do the next rep.

You can do reps on the same leg. You can alternate reps. Also try combining this with the rolling pistol for more fun.

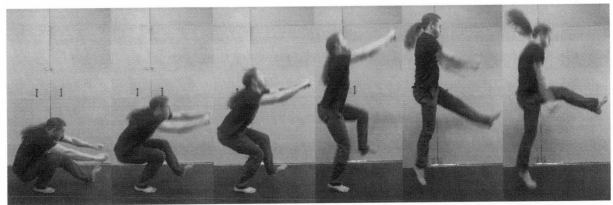

Go for maximum explosiveness out of the bottom and maximum height.

Box Jumping Pistols

In this version of the jumping pistol you add something to jump up onto. You can jump forwards, backwards and to the side. The side is the easiest and most comfortable one to do in my opinion.

Even a small height can be a challenge, especially if done for reps. You'll find that if you start going for a big height you'll end up coming up in the pistol but doing the jump with the last bit of your extension.

Make sure your surface is stable. I say this with personal experience. To see what happens when it's not safe and secure, check out this Jumping Pistol Blooper.
http://www.youtube.com/watch?v=okXtFP7fsGA

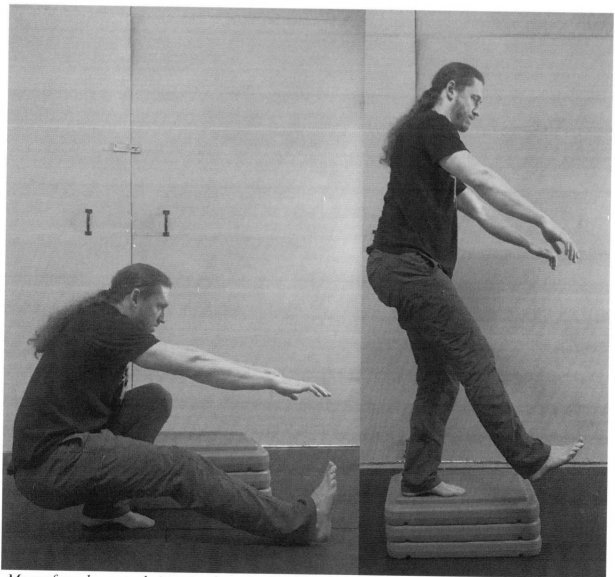

My preferred way to do jumping box pistols is to jump to the side of the leg you're squatting on.

Ball of Foot Pistol Squat

Some may call this a one-legged Hindu squat but usually the rowing arm motion is discarded with this as it interferes with the balance. A lot tougher than you might guess as all the bodyweight must be handled pretty much exclusively by the quadriceps.

Start in a standing position on one leg. Here the heel can be flat on the ground. But as you squat down, raise up on the toes with the free leg in front of you and a mostly upright back position. If you can pull off even one rep you're quite strong.

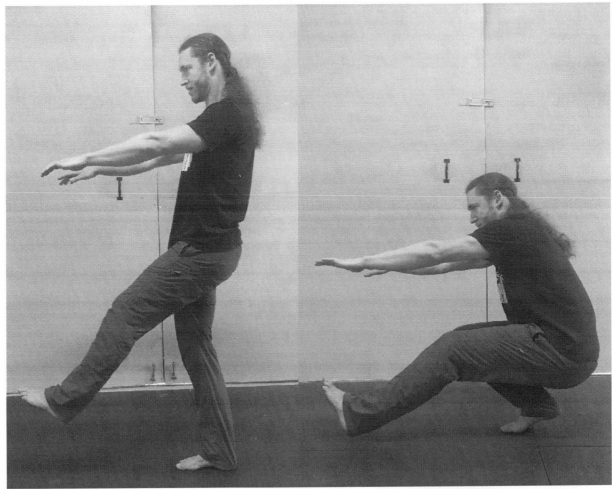

The more up on the ball of foot you are the more direct quad strength is required.

Weighted Pistols

As already discussed I am not a bodyweight purist. As was mentioned even the pistol can become an endurance test. But it's an easy move to add weight to to continually challenge your body. How you hold onto the weight will make some big changes.

With all these moves, as they change the center of gravity, the move will be slightly different in feel from a free pistol. If you have a heavy weight, or a light weight out far to counterbalance, then your weight can be fully on your heel rather than spread throughout your foot. At the same time, you can maintain a closer to upright back.

When it comes to weight, if you're lifting more than half your bodyweight in a pistol you're doing pretty good. Part of the Beast Challenge for men, originated with the RKC, is to do a pistol squat with a 48kg or 106 lb. kettlebell. The equivalent challenge for women, known as the Iron Maiden, is to do a pistol squat with a 24kg or 53 lb. kettlebell. These are good elite marks to shoot for.

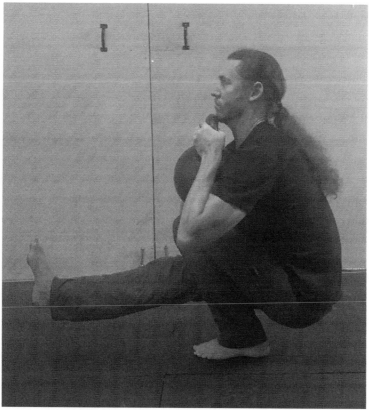

A pistol with the beast is a mighty mark for any man to shoot for.

One Weight Pistols

I typically use a kettlebell, but a dumbbell would work just as well. You can hold it by the horns or in the goblet position as you do the squat. Here it will also act as a counter weight. In fact, if you extend it further you can end up raising your butt then doing a good-morning-like-move rather than squatting out of the position.

I find this happens to me sometimes when I go for a max as my back is stronger than my legs. (From doing more deadlifts than weighted squats, as well as lots of kettlebell swings, snatches and juggling.) But not to worry, this can easily be minimized if it's a problem for you with the next version.

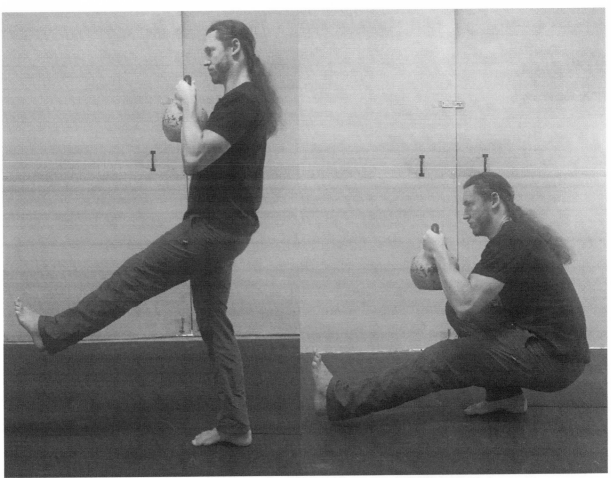

Holding a kettlebell by the horns for the pistol squat.
Here you can hold out the weight to act as a counterbalance, more so than in other styles.

One Weight in Rack Position Pistol

Instead of holding the weight out in front of you, hold it in the rack or cleaned position. Usually the weight will be held on the same side of the body as the leg that is squatting but you can do it on the opposite side. If you do your body will naturally rotate to some degree.

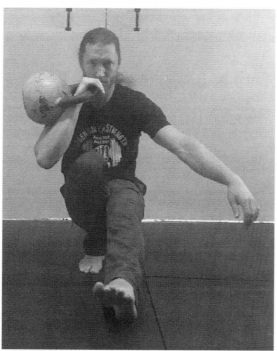

Racking the kettlebell on the same side as the squatting leg is a more natural position.

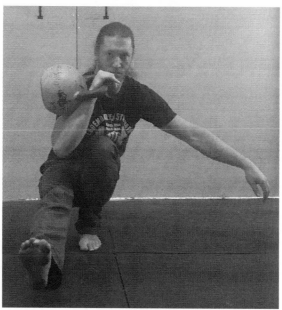

Notice the lean to the side to counter balance the weight in the opposite side rack position.

Two Weight Pistol

With two kettlebells or dumbbells in the rack position more of the weight will be centered over your foot. This allows you to work up to some big weights. Like the previous version you won't be able to lever out the weights and thus it will keep you in a stricter squat.

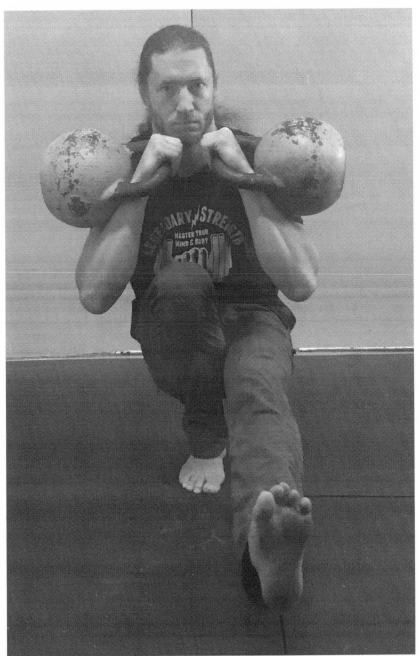

Holding onto two kettlebells is a natural position. Keep them even over your working leg.

Cable Pistols

An alternative to weights is to introduce the cable once again. Place the band over your shoulders and both the ends under your squatting foot. Note that this can be awkward as the cable may get in your way as you squat. For that reason alone, I prefer weights to cables in adding resistance to pistols.

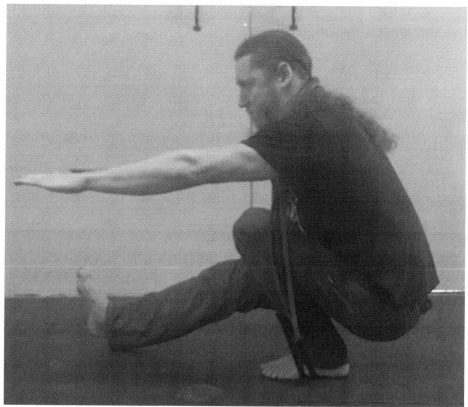

Don't want to mess with weights? Fine, you can add resistance with cables here too.

Weight Vest Pistols

The weight vest can also be used here. As the weight is more centered over your body and less in front of you as when you're holding weights, it is going to change the center of gravity, requiring more forward lean.

There's no reason you couldn't also combine the weight vest and holding kettlebells or other weights if your legs are strong enough to handle that much weight.

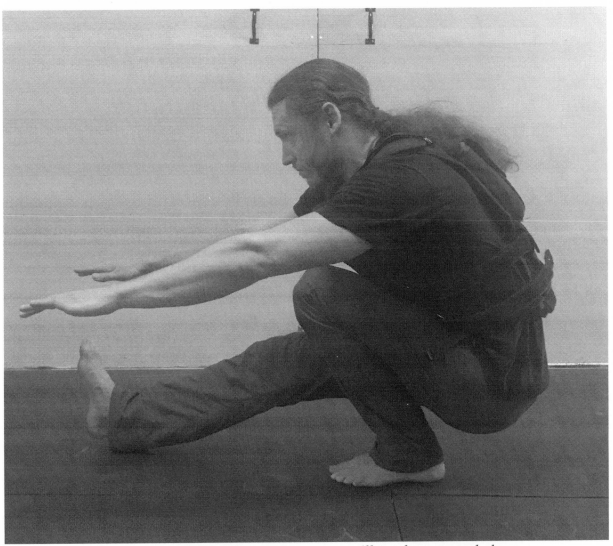

Note that with the weight on your torso you'll need to counterbalance by putting more of your weight forward.

How to Train to Rep Out Pistols

Occasionally, when I'm traveling or don't have lots of time to workout one of the things I do is a single all-out (or close to it) set of pistols on each leg. If you're getting in the 15-30 range or higher and you don't train these regularly, watch out! You'll likely find that you're quite sore the next day especially in the glutes. So, this can be a simple and effective workout to do occasionally.

But how should you train to increase your reps? The first step will be to figure out what your max is. If this is 2 reps or 20 this method can work for you. Cut that max number in half and this will be your working number.

One method is to do your working number throughout the day getting as many sets as you can do without getting fatigued or sore. This can be done daily or every other day with great success.

The same thing can be done in a single workout too. Just add to the number of sets you can do in a time frame and you'll get better.

With either of these methods occasionally add a rep to your working sets. After you've done this for 2 to 3 weeks give yourself two days of rest then max out again. If you don't find your new max higher you did something wrong! Go ahead and repeat this method once again until you reach the goal you're going for.

Once you get up to higher numbers of reps you may have to do a little less total volume. Be careful of doing too much if your sets are more than 12 reps each. At this point you're also getting to a place where once again achieving another rep is mental toughness and you may be able to power through all the way to 50 reps.

My friend once held a contest at his gym with pistols. The winner got some big prize. The numbers were staggering with the winner doing 123 pistols on one leg! Sometimes having a big incentive is all you need.

If you can learn to stand on your one leg and rest a bit before the next pistol, you'll be able to do more and more reps. Seldom are these long sets done without some rest in the top position.

How to Train to Add Weight to Pistols

A similar workout program as that done to add reps will work for adding weight to pistols. Choose a weight that you can do a few reps with and then work about half that number consistently.

Because of the nature of the pistol I've found it's not something you want to do maxing out on very much. Your position can tend to break down as you struggle with a max weight. Instead it is much better to work with weights you can handle for at least a few reps at a time.

You can still max it out when you choose to I just wouldn't recommend a program of heavy singles.

5x5

A five by five program would also work well for this move twice a week. After two warmup sets select your working weight. Aim to hit 3 sets of 5 on each leg with this weight. Then for the next workout add a little bit of weight. (If you're working with kettlebells don't be jumping 4 or especially 8 kilograms at a time. Try smaller jumps like two pounds and you'll make better progress.)

For example:

1. Warmup set Bodyweight only x 5 reps each leg
2. Warmup set 16kg x 5 reps each leg
3. Working set 24kg x 5 reps each leg
4. Working set 24kg x 5 reps each leg
5. Working set 24kg x 5 reps each leg

If you hit the three sets of five with your working weight, then in the next workout you would add more.

Waving Weights and Volume (includes Explosive Pistols)

Another option is to vary the weight you use from a workout to workout basis. For instance, I might do bodyweight pistols one workout, 16kg the next, 32kg the following, then back to bodyweight, this time explosive ones.

Increase what you can do at each of these points and you'll see improvements in them all. Strive for higher max reps in each set and/or total volume you do.

Workout 1
Bodyweight pistols x 10/10, 8/8, 8/8, 5/5 = 62 total reps

(This is read as 10 reps left, 10 reps right, 8 reps left, 8 reps right, and so on.)

Workout 2
16kg pistols x 6/6, 5/5, 5/5 = 32 total reps

Workout 3
32kg pistols x 1/1, 2/2, 3/3 = 12 total reps

Workout 4
Jumping bodyweight pistols x 5/5, 5/5, 4/4 = 28 total reps

The jumping pistols can be done as box jumps or simply jumping pistols depending on whichever you want to do.

As before, chances are that your legs aren't exactly equal, so there's a good chance your workouts may look more like this:

Workout 1
Bodyweight pistols x 10/12, 7/8, 6/8, 5/6 = 62 total reps

Workout 2
24kg pistols x 5/6, 4/5, 3/5 = 28 total reps

And so on.

Improving Flexibility and Mobility Pistol Plan

Working with the various extra bodyweight versions of pistols will help you to deepen your flexibility and mobility even further. This workout is a good one to try before moving onto the next module, or as you begin to train the other one-legged squats.

But don't think this is just an easy flexibility and mobility workout. Especially as the explosive movements come into play you'll find this is a great explosive workout too.

- Switching Legs x 20 alternating
- Sit to Pistol x 20 alternating
- Ball of Foot Pistol x 20 alternating
- Cossack Dance (flat footed) x 20 alternating
- Cossack Dance (ball of foot) x 20 alternating
- Box Jumping x 4 sets of 5 each leg

Module 6 – Other One-Legged Squats

For years I thought that the pistol squat was the king of lower body leg exercises. In fact, I knew only of it and wasn't aware of these other one-legged squats. But then, a few years ago, learning from Al and Danny Kavadlo I was exposed to several other variations worth doing…and worth mastering.

The added challenge of the shrimp squat, figure 4 squat and dragon pistol squat steps up how difficult bodyweight leg training can be. These require even greater levels of active flexibility and mobility than the pistol. As you're just squatting your bodyweight, the strength demands aren't really any higher, except that you need to exert that strength in flexible positions.

For that reason, everything discussed so far regarding building strength from bodyweight leg training is still true. But for the elite bodyweight man or woman this offers a variety of new challenges to take you even deeper.

When I started practicing these I figured a good challenge was to then sequence the four different one-legged squats together, as they each put the free leg in a different direction. That is:

Pistol – Front
Dragon Pistol – Inside
Shrimp – Rear
Figure 4 – Outside

Thus, you go "around the clock," which gives you what I call the 4-Way One Legged Squat, a difficult challenge worth finishing this book with.

Airborne Lunge

The airborne lunge is a version of the one-legged squat that is easier than the classic pistol and serves as a preliminary move to the shrimp squat.

Keep your free leg bent behind you as you squat down. Your arms and torso will still be leaning forward too. The knee of the free leg touches the ground and then you come back up. Your heel must remain planted throughout the range of motion.

Because the free leg is behind you, your working leg can maintain more of an upright position. This reduces the flexibility demands, allowing you to work the strength of the one leg, without what turns out to be a limiting factor for many people. It is similar to the elevated pistol squat covered earlier in this respect.

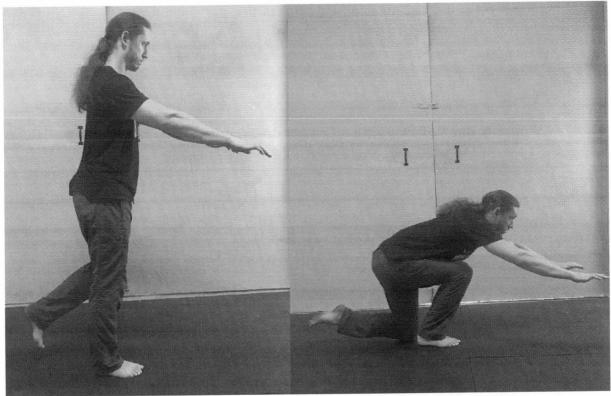

Lean far forward to reach your torso to your thigh.

Weighted Airborne Lunge

In *Ultimate Athleticism*, Max Shank discusses this as one of four exercises worth doing that basically covers all the strength you need (in addition to the deadlift, front lever, and L-press to handstand.) https://amzn.to/2NRENGR

And there is good reason for the choice of this move over the weighted pistol. In general, it is just a bit more user friendly. Excessive amounts of volume, or with weights, in pistols may not work for a whole lot of people considering the amount of knee issues that abound. Meanwhile, the airborne lunge delivers pretty much the same benefits with lower risk and without the same flexibility demands.

One or two kettlebells or dumbbells. You can try all the kettlebell positions mentioned earlier but holding one by the horns will be the most natural here.

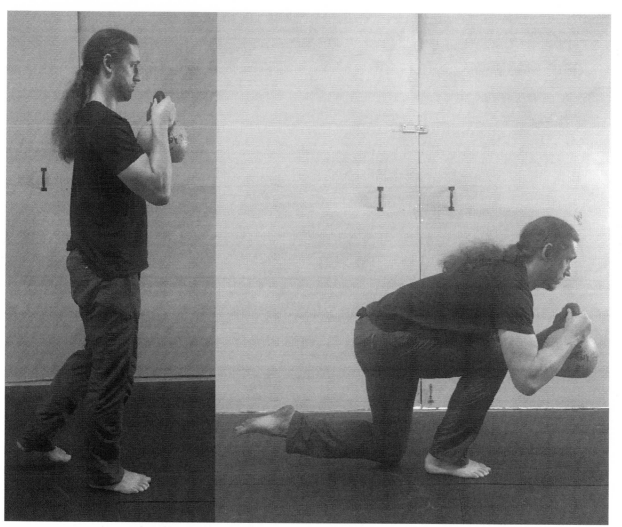

A weighted airborne lunge using one kettlebell for added resistance.

Zercher Airborne Lunge

When using a barbell, you'll want to use the Zercher position, named after St. Louis strongman Ed Zercher from back in the 1930s and later. This position involves holding the barbell in the crooks of your elbows. While this may be uncomfortable at first, with a little practice you'll get used to it.

It is easiest to grab the bar from a rack rather than from the ground when in the position, although it can be grabbed from the ground.

You can also do the airborne lunge with the barbell on the shoulder but the Zercher is a bit more fun.

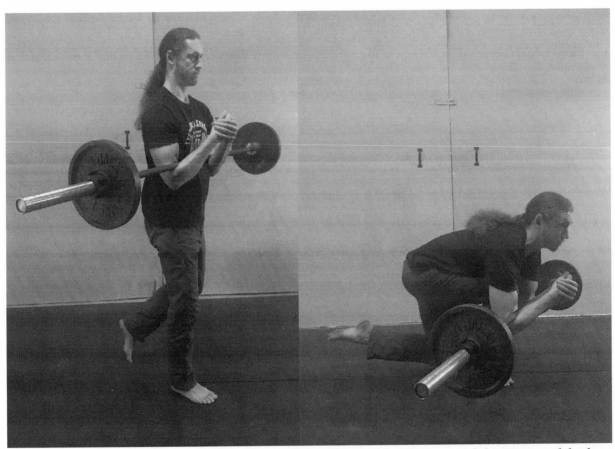

It may look odd, but with a little practice you'll get use to this position and this is one of the best ways to build great one-legged strength.

Shrimp Squat

If you can easily do the airborne lunge than you may be ready for the shrimp squat. The position is the same except that the same side arm as the free leg grabs onto the foot. Your other arm, the same side as the working leg, will come forward to act as a counterbalance.

Work to find the best holding position of the free foot for you. I do a thumbless grip over the top of the toes.

This requires flexibility in the hip flexor area of the free leg to allow you to descend to a bottom position. In addition, the working leg needs stronger dorsiflexion to keep the hips over the working foot.

Be careful that the working foot's heel stays planted the entire time. If you're coming up on your toes this is an indicator that you've reached the limits of your current flexibility. While you can choose to do ball of foot shrimp squats, the true shrimp squat is flat footed.

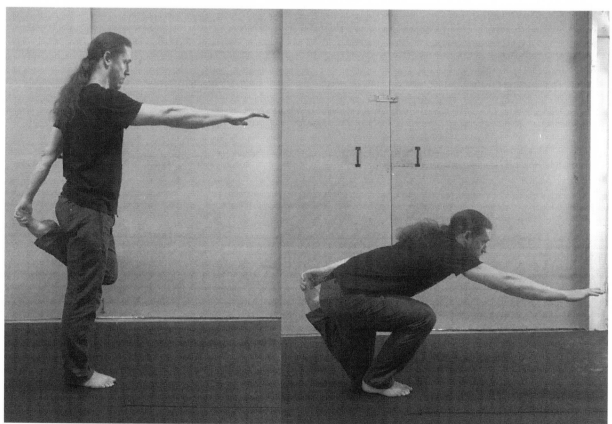

Holding onto your leg with one or both arms increases the difficulty significantly.

Shrimp Squat Hand and Foot Position

These two pictures show you a close up of how I hold onto my foot for the shrimp squat and the double shrimp squat. You may find a better position for yourself, but these have worked best for me. (Forgive the dirty feet, that's what happens on these rubber mats I work on.)

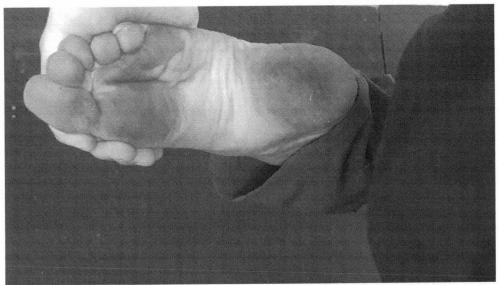

The same side hand cups over the shrimp foot in the shrimp squat.

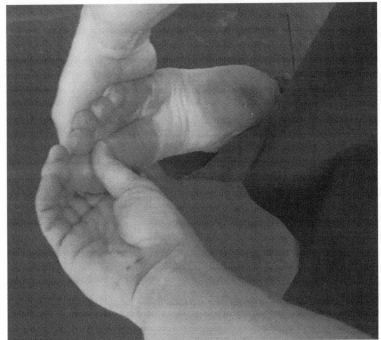

In the double shrimp squat, the same side hand takes the same position as before, except the pinkie is less around the big toe. That's because the opposite side hand grabs onto that big toe.

Double Shrimp Squat

For the double shrimp squat, both hands are reaching behind you and grabbing the free leg by the foot. I typically grab the big toe by the hand that is the same side as the working leg. The other hand is still a thumbless grip over the toes, but only four of the toes now instead of them all.

Because both hands are reaching behind the flexibility demands increase much further. Now you do not have even one arm to counterbalance your weight forward. This means even more of an upright position along with increased dorsiflexion is required.

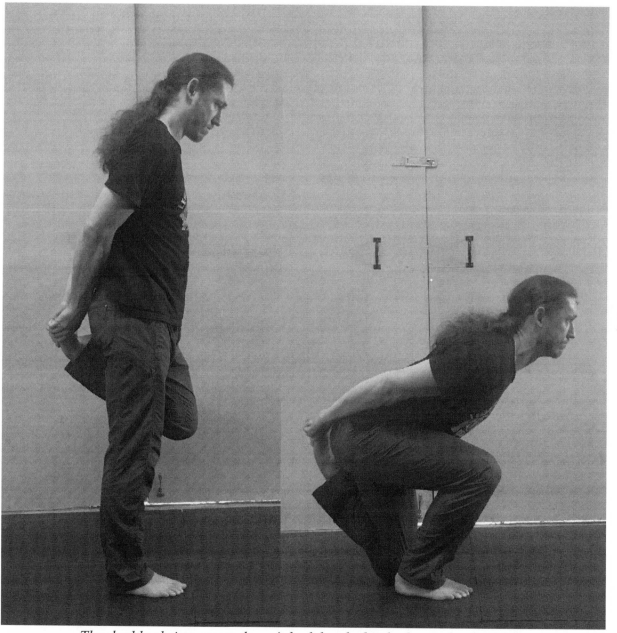

The double shrimp squat doesn't look hard...but looks can be deceiving.

Range of Motion in Shrimp Squats

The best way to progress with the airborne lunge, shrimp and double shrimp squats is by extending the range of motion over time. What this means is that you put the boxes, or rather I find smaller increments like skinny phonebooks, under the free knee. Here you won't have to go down as far and thus it is easier to do. Then, like before, you work on extending the range of motion as you progress.

This method works best when combined with targeting stretching of the hip flexors and ankle as needed.

You can use this first with the airborne lunge, then move onto the shrimp squat and then move onto the double shrimp squat as a progression through the increasing difficulty of these moves.

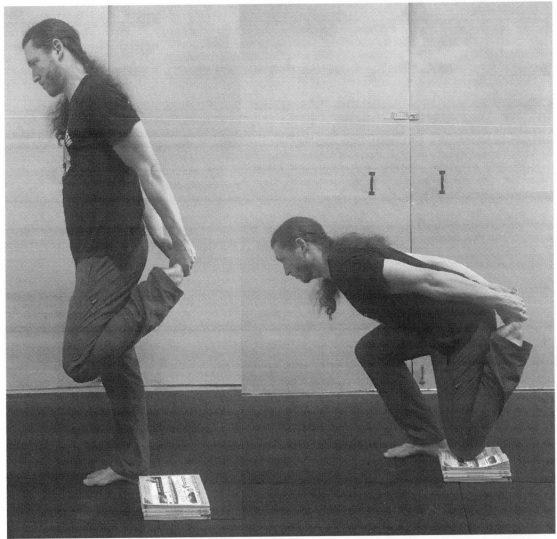

While shown with the double shrimp squat, this method applies to the regular shrimp too, and even the airborne lunge if you need it there.

Jumbo Shrimp Squat

We can take what we were doing before in extending range of motion to complete the full shrimp exercise and take it even further.

Progress in the exact same way as before just a fraction of an inch at a time. Start with the jumbo shrimp squat and once you've attained a true full range of motion on this, that is rock bottom where your thigh rests on your calf, then you can begin to train the double jumbo shrimp squat. In other words, start with the one hand, and when you are ready move to both hands.

Note that this takes increasingly crazy amounts of hip flexor flexibility, without any more dorsiflexion.

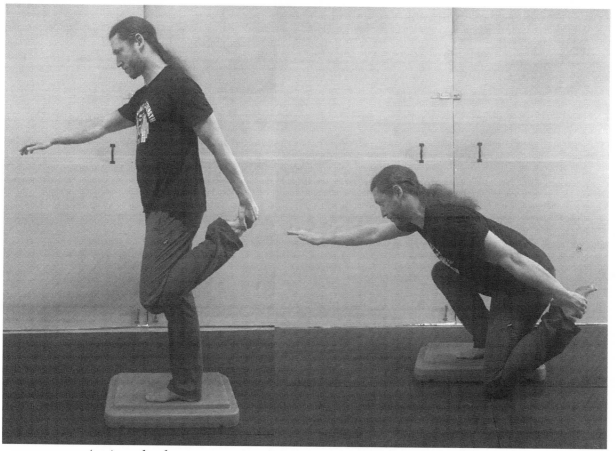

Again, take the progress in moving into the jumbo shrimp squat slowly.

Figure 4 Squat

The figure 4 squat is also known as the Hawaiian squat. I prefer the figure 4 name as it is more descriptive and doesn't lock you into a location. The top position takes the free leg, rotates it to the outside, with the lower leg coming across and resting over the knee of the working leg. It looks like a "4," hence the name.

Be forewarned that when you first start working on this it can be uncomfortable on the working knee. Not only are your squatting your whole bodyweight, which your likely used to at this point, but having the free leg resting on it exerts a downward pressure on the muscles seemingly causing them to fire somewhat differently. For this reason, ease into this slowly.

Again, as in all one-legged squats, we have increased dorsiflexion demands. And here we also have external hip rotation flexibility needed for the first time. Added stretching in these areas can assist in progression.

If your flexibility is limited, you'll likely be stopped up somewhere around parallel, being unable to go lower without falling backwards. But ideally, we want to get into a rock bottom squat, that is thigh on calf.

Note that if you cannot get into the bottom position even while holding onto an object you'll need to work on your basic flexibility more before training this move.

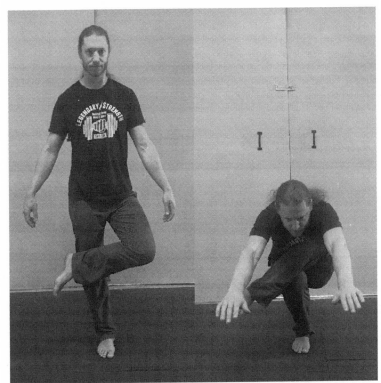

I'm still developing flexibility for this. Other people may be able to hold the figure 4 in more of a lotus-like position.

Figure 4 Squat Hold

Extending range of motion didn't work as well in this exercise like it did in others. The limiting factor seems to be in counterbalancing your own weight, which is why we use that to progress.

In the beginning, holding onto a static object will allow you to pull yourself all the way down. Get used to this position even holding for time. Try to counter less of your weight with your hands over time. I like to hold this for 30 seconds to a minute long.

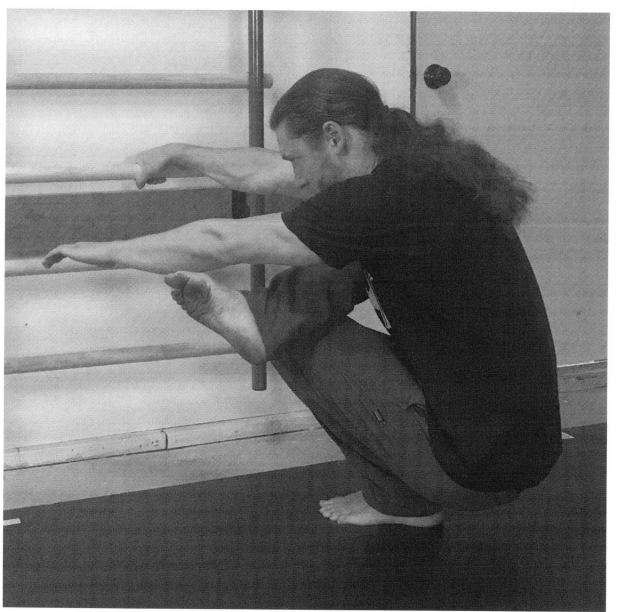

Strive to relax into this position, and over time, pull less with your hands.

Counterbalanced Figure 4 Squat

Then we move onto using light weights to act as a counterbalance. I like to start with 10 lbs. then move down. This includes using 5 lbs., 2½ lbs., and 1¼ lbs. Get into a rock bottom figure 4 squat with each of these then you're reading to start doing bodyweight only with the full range.

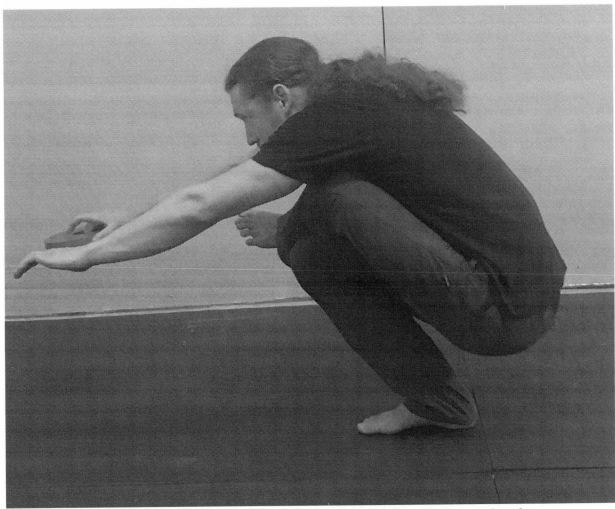

Note the lower position achieved by holding a 5 lb. plate in one hand.

Dragon Pistol

The dragon pistol is one of the coolest looking one-legged squat moves. It's also somewhat confusing the first time you try it. The free leg wraps around and underneath the working leg, requiring a good amount of active flexibility to hold it up off the ground.

In addition to stretching your arms forward so that you don't fall backwards, since the free leg is going slightly out to the side, you also need to lean your torso away from that leg. Also pay attention to the fact that you can get the leg fully extended, but still not be quite in the rock-bottom position.

As you become used to the position you can use your hands on the floor to help you find the balance. Simply holding the bottom position of the dragon pistol is a useful way to build up the ability. This is the hardest part, though transferring into and out of this position is not so easy either.

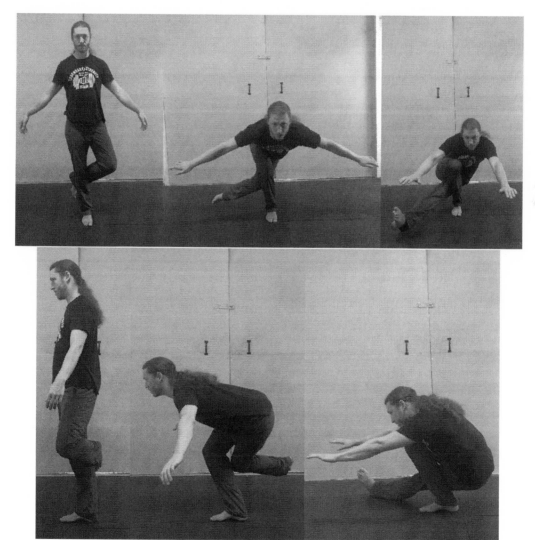

Notice the aggressive forward lean as the rear leg sweeps through in the middle of the move.

Assisted Dragon Pistol

The best way to get started in doing the dragon pistol is to do the assisted dragon pistol. In this you use the opposite side arm to grab onto the free leg. I find it best to just grab onto the big toe, though you may find a different position that is more comfortable to you.

You hold onto the foot for the entire movement. This means you start out with the knee bent and behind you, kind of like a reverse figure-4. By holding onto the foot, you can support the active flexibility that is needed in helping to keep it aloft.

Get good at the assisted dragon pistol, while also working on regular dragon pistol holds in the bottom position and you should be able to accomplish the full move in no time.

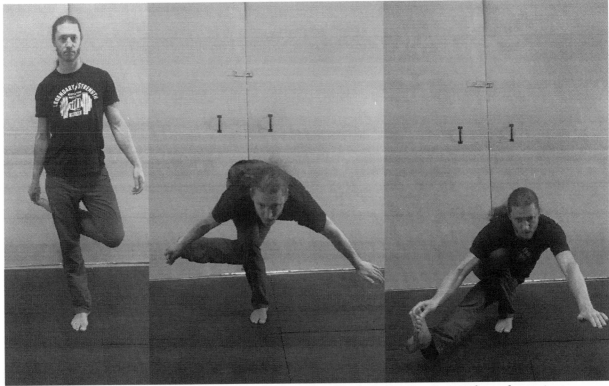

Having that hand hold onto your foot makes the dragon pistol significantly easier.

4 Way One-Legged Squat

Different people may find that one of the four variations of the one-legged squats is harder than another. This depends on your flexibility and which places may hold you back more so than others.

In any case, over time you'll want to work on them all. But more focus should go into your weak spots. Eventually, you can put them together for this elite level move.

I typically do them in the following order: pistol, dragon pistol, double shrimp, figure 4. That being said, you can do the reverse or mix them up however you like.

Just getting a full rep in each one of these back to back is great. And then you can do reps. Two reps would be two full cycles through, so eight one-legged squats. Three reps would be twelve squats and so on.

The great thing about this move is that once you have it, by combining it in this manner, it should be fairly easy to maintain and expand upon.

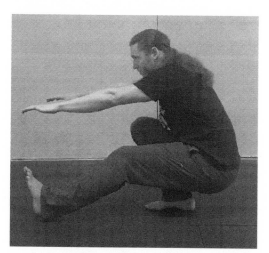
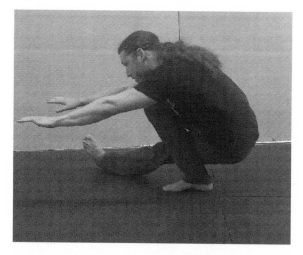

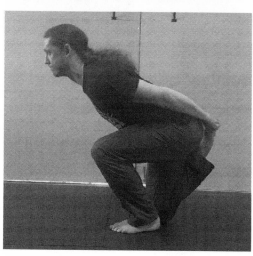
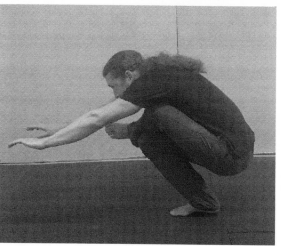

Training the Four One-Legged Squats

The concepts and even training plans covered before can be adapted to any of these moves. Specifically, what was covered in the previous chapters on pistols will be useful here.

In addition to that, what follows are some additional tips and training ideas that will allow you to focus more on achieving and expanding on the moves in this module.

Achieving the Shrimp Squat and Beyond

Recall that there is a progression just in these moves:

1. Airborne Lunge
2. Shrimp Squat
3. Double Shrimp Squat
4. Jumbo Shrimp Squat
5. Double Jumbo Shrimp Squat

(Both double shrimp and jumbo shrimp could be worked at the same time, in parallel progressions, but it could just as easily be done linearly as laid out.)

What follows applies to any of these variations, though I'll just say shrimp squats to keep it simple.

Follow the same steps as far as progressing with box squats or box pistols, just in this case you'll want smaller jumps, around ½" or so. Once again, I like to use a stack of skinny phonebooks for this purpose. Your knee touches down to this stack, so you work on progressing range of motion.

Once you get to the jumbo shrimp squats, you start standing on this elevated stack with your knee touching the ground.

Day 1
Max depth 6"
3 sets of 10 reps each leg at 7.5"

Day 2
5 sets of 12 reps each leg at 8"

Day 3
8 sets of 15 reps each leg at 9"

Day 4
4 sets of 6 reps each leg at 7"

Day 5
8 sets of 20 reps each leg at 8.5"

Day 6
6 sets of 3 reps each leg at 6.5"

Day 6
5 sets of 20 reps each leg at 8"

Day 7
8 sets of 2 reps each leg at 6"

Day 8
New max depth at 5"
3 sets of 6 reps each leg at 6"

Achieving the Figure 4 Squat

Here, range of motion as a progression doesn't work as well. Instead using counterbalancing weight seems to work better.

Supported Bottom Position Figure 4 Hold x 30 seconds each leg
Counterbalance Figure 4 Squat + 20 lbs. x 3-6 each leg
Counterbalance Figure 4 Squat + 10 lbs. x 3-6 each leg
Counterbalance Figure 4 Squat + 5 lbs. x 3-6 each leg
Counterbalance Figure 4 Squat + 2.5 lbs. x 3-6 each leg
Counterbalance Figure 4 Squat + 1.25 lbs. x 3-6 each leg
Counterbalance Figure 4 Squat + 0.5 lbs. x 3-6 each leg
Counterbalance Figure 4 Squat Full x 3-6 each leg

You can do this workout each day. The hold in the beginning serves as a useful warmup.

After that, only go as far as you feel you can get to the bottom position. Don't allow the heel to come up. If that happens, or you just can't go further down, use a larger weight. In the beginning 10 lbs. may be as far as you get, so you stop there (potentially doing a few extra sets with that weight).

But as you progress you should be able to handle it with less and less counterweight. If you don't have small weight plates you can use something like a book that is approximately that weight.

I find that doing at least three reps helps to get the groove better and allow you to progress more so than just doing a rep at a time. Pausing in the bottom of the squat also helps rather than bouncing in and out of it quickly.

Achieving the Dragon Pistol

Neither range of motion, nor counterbalancing worked all that well for progressing with the dragon pistol. Instead, training the bottom position and then using the assisted version was enough. Thus, how to train for these looks a little different.

Assisted Dragon Pistol Bottom Position Hold – Build up to 30 seconds each leg
Assisted Dragon Pistol – Build up to 20 each leg
Dragon Pistol Bottom Position Hold – Build up to 30 seconds each leg
Dragon Pistol – Build up to 20 each leg

Previously when I mentioned the hold you might have thought to start that just with the full dragon pistol position. But this can also be done in the assisted version. Because it is such an uncommon position just about everyone will have to start here. If you cannot hold the bottom assisted position, work more on your basic flexibility before pursuing this move. But if you can hold it you're good to start.

As with all things you're likely to find one leg is better than the other. It is not just a test of flexibility but of balance too. Work several sets of the holds. At some point it is likely to "click" and you'll start progressing much faster, even finding 30 seconds easy.

Once you have reached 30 seconds in the assisted hold, begin to work on the unassisted hold. If you need to you can do an intermediary step of assisting, but less so. That is pull your foot up less with your hand, making that free leg do more of the work.

Parallel to working the holds, you want to work on the full motion. The bottom position is the toughest part but getting into and out of it isn't so easy either. You want to train both.

Buildup in reps what you can do with the assisted dragon pistol. By the time you can do twenty reps per leg you should be able to do at least one unassisted dragon pistol. Then start building from there.

Achieving All at Once

You will make more progress in these squats if you devote more time to them one at a time. More frequency of training will help build the skill, balance and flexibility needed.

In my own training I had done this and achieved them all before. But then my training went another direction and I stopped working on them. When I wanted to regain them, I started working on them all at once. I did this with one dedicated session to each of the four one-legged squats once per week. In a way each one supports at least some of the ability you need in the others, but not fully. While I did get there, I know that it was slower than if I had done more frequent training.

But once you've achieved them all you can put them together and use the 4-way one-legged squat as your method of training and progression. My current training involves four sessions a week where I work on the 4-way move as well as a bit more targeted work where I feel I need it.

Build up to doing 10 reps of the 4-way (which equals a total of 40 one-legged squats) and you've got some amazing leg strength, endurance and flexibility.

30 Minutes One Leg Squat Challenge

What if we took that concept of the 30-minute squat challenge from the very first module and elevated it to an elite level? Enter the 30 minute one-leg squat challenge. This could be done with any single variation…or by mixing and matching the four versions.

For the pistol squat, dragon pistol and figure 4 squat the bottom position is self-explanatory.

But not so much for the shrimp squat. Here, since your knee would be on the ground, we'll want to instead use the rock-bottom position of a jumbo shrimp, where the knee is free-hanging. This is going to take very flexible hip flexors.

As before, it's not to do 30 minutes straight. But to do half a minute, one minute, two minutes here and there throughout your day. If you can accomplish this with the one-legged squats you're doing something far beyond most people's abilities.

Appendix A
Ultimate Bodyweight Program Template

How do you combine different bodyweight exercises together in order to cover the whole body? That is what this report is all about.

More specifically, how do you use bodyweight exercises to continually build strength and conditioning across your body from rank beginner to elite levels?

To the average trainee out there, bodyweight exercises only means such calisthenics as pushups, bodyweight squats and situps. They have no clue about countless variations available and even less about how to progressively train with those variations.

I call this the Ultimate Bodyweight Program TEMPLATE for a reason. It is not so much a program in that I lay out every single detail for you. I don't know which exercises you know. I don't know what your current strength is across these different exercises. I don't know your goals. And I don't know your body, with its inherent strengths and weaknesses, possible injuries and what-have-you.

For these reasons, I can't give you a cookie-cutter program that will work for you specifically. But what I can deliver is a simple yet effective template that you can easily adapt to your current level and your own needs. **And if you understand this template it could serve you for years to come!**

Over my career as a strongman and trainer, I have used this template and recommended it to others. It works because it builds your foundational strength in the necessary areas of the human body. The template works generally. Then it is up to you to plug into it the specific exercises for where you're at. Add a bit of work and voila, you will get results.

When I originally got into bodyweight training I was focused on higher rep stuff. Sets of fifty or a hundred reps were not uncommon. Sometimes I went even higher. But as I continued training I found greater benefits on focusing more on strength than endurance. **Those sets of five reps worked better than fifty.** Even singles and doubles had their place!

This high-strength bodyweight training was a different approach than most took. (Some people say that bodyweight training is only good for endurance. Well, that's just because they don't know the right variations to progress to these strength levels.)

It was in playing with some of these high-strength bodyweight exercises that I originally stumbled upon what I named the "Fearless Foursome Workout." This took what I saw as the best bodyweight exercises and grouped them together. The exercises from this workout is what started the whole *Ultimate Guide to Bodyweight Training Series* in the first place. The four exercises were:

1. Handstand Pushup
2. Pullup
3. Pistol Squat
4. Hanging Leg Raise

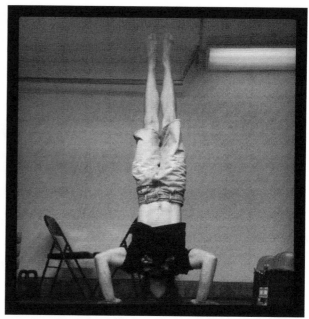

And that is the essence of the Template. But you may be saying, "I can't do all those exercises!" I get that. I couldn't do any of them when I started training either.

For example, it took me about six months of dedicated training before I accomplished my first handstand pushup. Nowadays I'm doing full range and freestanding handstand pushups. **If I could do it, the possibility is open for you.**

So don't worry, that is just one example of the template in action…

The Template

That above example is what I would call an intermediate level of exercises in the template. To generalize it, what the template really looks like is the following:

1. Upper body pushing exercise
2. Upper body pulling exercise
3. Lower body squat exercise
4. Ab exercise

To give you more examples of what this will look like, here is a beginner level of exercises:

1. Pushup
2. Inverted Row
3. Basic Squat
4. V-up

And an insanely strong and advanced level:

1. Full range freestanding handstand pushups
2. One arm chin-ups
3. 4-way one legged squats
4. Standing ab wheel rollouts

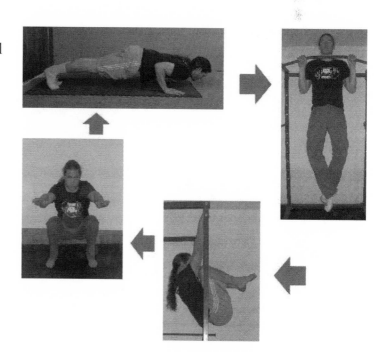

The template stands as it is, it just becomes a matter of doing the variations that are suitable for your level of strength. This brings us to the next section…

Exercise Selection

Going into the details of the following list of exercises is beyond the scope of this report. For more details please see *The Ultimate Bodyweight Training Series*, which is broken up across the specific types of exercise.

You can also just launch YouTube and enter in the name of the exercise there (though I can't speak to the quality of instruction you're likely to find).

The following lists are not exhaustive, meaning I'm not listing out every possible variation of exercise there is. What I have found is that **often times people get lost in variations rather than recognizing that progression is the name of the game.** For that reason, I list these in approximate degree of difficulty, though sometimes there are parallel tracks.

Upper body pushing exercises
- Wall pushup
- Knee pushup
- Incline pushup
- Regular pushup
- Decline pushup
- Hindu pushup
- Dive bomber pushup
- Hand-on-hand pushup
- Pike press
- Handstand shrugs
- Partial handstand pushup
- Easy handstand pushup
- Medium handstand pushup
- Hard handstand pushup
- Increased ROM handstand pushup
- Full range handstand pushup
- Freestanding handstand pushup
- Tiger bend
- Full range freestanding handstand pushup
- One arm handstand pushup

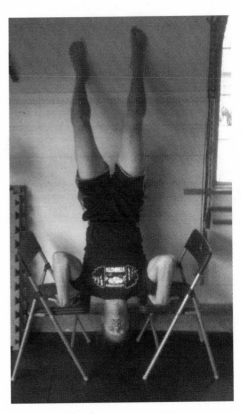

Upper body pulling exercise

- Angled inverted row
- Inverted row knees bent
- Inverted row straight legs
- Chin-up hold

- Chin-up negative
- Partial chin-up
- Regular chin-up
- Pullup
- Weighted pullup
- Muscle up
- Archer pullup
- One arm assisted chin-up
- One arm chin-up
- One arm pullup

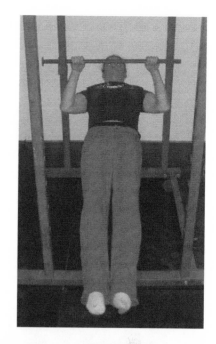

Lower body squat exercise

- Basic squat
- Hindu squat
- Rollback squat
- Split stance squat
- Lunge
- Circular squat
- Side to side squat
- Jump squat
- Airborne lunge
- Pistol squat
- Jumping pistol squat
- Shrimp squat
- Double shrimp squat
- Jumbo shrimp squat
- Figure 4 squat
- Assisted dragon pistol squat
- Dragon pistol squat
- 4-way one legged squat

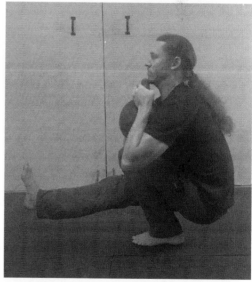

Ab exercise

- Crunch
- Situp
- V-up
- N-sit
- L-sit
- V-sit
- Hanging knee raises
- Hanging leg raises
- One arm hanging leg raises
- Knee ab wheel rollouts
- Standing incline ab wheel rollouts
- Standing ab wheel rollouts

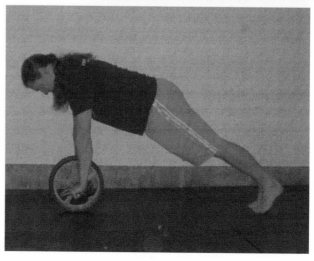

- One leg standing ab wheel rollouts
- Weighted standing ab wheel rollouts

As you can see **there are variations for the frailest of the frail, up to the strongest of the strong. The key is in progressing from one end to the other.**

Also note that there are variations within the variations. An incline pushup is not one exercise but a wide degree of angles that can be used, making the progressive steps so small as to be unnoticeable if so desired. The one arm assisted chin-up has many steps or levels that can be used, which by itself could take a year of training to move through. Once again, the details of these are beyond the scope of this report but can be found in detail inside the *Ultimate Guides*.

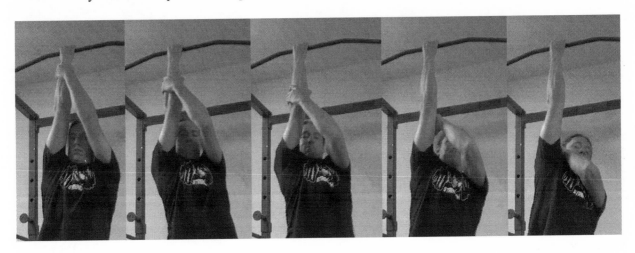

Sets and Reps

We've covered the template. We've covered the exercises to do. The next question is how many reps and sets should you do? There is one and only one answer.

4 sets of 6 reps.

...just kidding.

There is no magic set and rep scheme. You can do one set to failure. You can do ten sets of easy low reps. You can do twenty sets of thirteen reps if you want. Once again, the key is progression, not some specific amount of volume. This means that whatever you do in training, do better than last time (volume, or the number of sets and reps being just one way of doing better.)

Four sets of six reps can work very well, but it is far from the only option. I'd say in general somewhere between one and ten sets is going to work for you. You can do one or two sets but if you do you'll need to work harder on each one of them. In general, at least three sets is best if you're not going towards your limit i.e. training to failure.

And on the other side, if you're doing more than ten sets you probably should have gone with something harder to begin with. You can go beyond this range, but in general somewhere between one to ten sets is good, with at least three sets being best.

As for reps you want to aim for somewhere between three and twenty reps. You can do singles and doubles, but generally I find doing a few more reps gives you more practice in the movement as well as a greater training effect. In my opinion, singles are more for testing your strength than building it. (I say that despite really loving to do singles myself!)

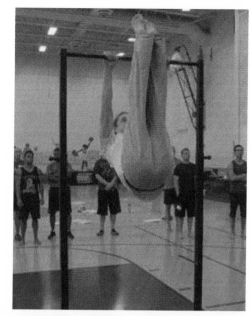

On the other end, **I find that twenty reps is a good upper limit for a strength exercise**. Beyond that you're getting into endurance territory (well, strength-endurance really). Lately, I've considered myself "graduated" from an exercise variation once I can do a set of twenty reps in it. Once here, I move on up to the next difficulty progression.

One key difference here is with squats. As the leg muscles are stronger, especially when it comes to two-legged squats, you can go up to sets of 50. Once you start doing one-legged squats, then the rep range of 3-20 becomes appropriate again. But with two legged squats it makes sense to go higher.

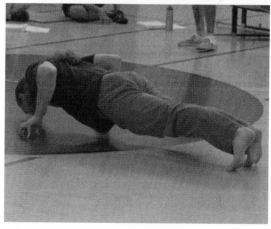

You can go outside all these numbers, just understand why I put them here in the first place. Thus, to add our sets and reps to the template it looks like this:

1. Upper Body Push Variation x 1-10 sets x 3-20 reps
2. Upper Body Pull Variation x 1-10 sets x 3-20 reps
3. Squat Variation x 1-10 sets x 3-50 reps
4. Ab Variation x 1-10 sets x 3-20 reps

You will be doing these in circuit fashion. That means you do one set of the upper body push, one set of the upper body pull, one set of the squat then one set of the ab exercise. Then you start back again at the upper body push and the cycle repeats for however many sets you're doing.

This is quite the range isn't it? One set of three reps is very, very different than ten sets of twenty! Understand, the purpose of this is to not get locked into a certain set and rep scheme.

What I want you to do is sometimes go lower volume with more difficult variations and sometimes go higher volume with easier variations. **I find that waving the volume and load makes is less likely that you'll get stuck at a plateau of doing the same thing over and over again.**

What follows are two examples of different workouts with different exercises selection and different sets and reps, but both are appropriate for approximately the same strength level using the template.

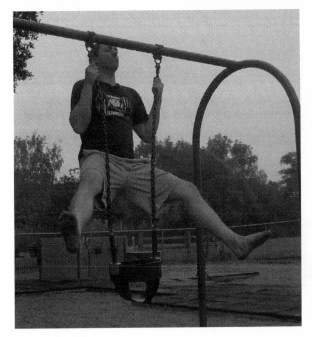

Lower Intensity/Higher Volume Workout
1.   Decline Pushup x 8 sets of 15 reps
2.   Chin-up x 8 sets of 6 reps
3.   Hindu Squat x 8 sets of 40 reps
4.   Hanging Knee Raise x 8 sets of 15 reps

Higher Intensity/Lower Volume Workout
1.   Medium Handstand Pushups x 4 sets of 3 reps
2.   Weighted Pullup with 35lbs. x 4 sets of 5 reps
3.   Jumping Pistol Squat x 4 sets of 5 reps each leg
4.   Full Hanging Leg Raise x 4 sets of 6 reps

Neither of these workouts is "better" than the other, they're just slightly differently focused.

What about Conditioning?

I find that strength is the main attribute of athleticism that the average person is best to focus on. Yes, you want the other ones. You want endurance, flexibility, mobility, balance, coordination and all the rest. But in focusing first and foremost on strength you can hit many of the other attributes.

Aiming for handstand pushups, pullups, pistols and hanging leg raises will give you an above average degree of flexibility, mobility, balance and coordination, especially as compared to the average, un-trained individual. You can add more work specifically on these other attributes if you so choose, but this template will at least provide a base.

But conditioning is important, and with the template, easily achieved. If these exercises are done in a circuit fashion, with as little rest as you can, you'll find that your cardiovascular system and breath is working harder than it would in running for miles! This is especially true with the higher volume workouts.

Since you're doing strength work, this is building both your anaerobic and aerobic capabilities to some degree. Many people only focus on their aerobic ability to the exclusion of anaerobic, when anaerobic is more important. (It also tends to carry over to the other, but not vice versa,

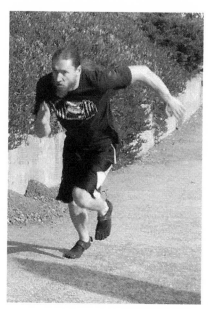

meaning that anaerobic training builds aerobic ability, but aerobic training does not build anaerobic ability).

If you want to focus more on strength, aim for higher intensity and lower reps. If this is the case you can rest for one to three minutes between exercises, keeping a leisurely pace. The "Higher Intensity/Lower Volume Workout" shown above is a good example of that.

If you want it to be more conditioning focused, up the rep count and aim to do it non-stop, or with as little rest as possible. This way you're getting strength and cardiovascular work at the same time. The "Lower Intensity/Higher Volume Workout" is a prime example of this.

And you can always add to the template with something like hill sprints, if you so choose. But it's not necessary.

Frequency of Training

The simplest way to do the Ultimate Bodyweight Template is as a single workout, meaning you're doing all four exercises in each workout. Many people will find that this can be done three times per week. (If you go more intense and/or higher volume in the workout, then twice a week may be sufficient. If you go easier than you may be able to do it four times per week. Recovery ability also changes from person to person.)

This template could also be split up so that you do shorter but more frequent workouts. One workout focuses on the upper body push and upper body pull. The other workout focuses on the squat and ab exercises. So…

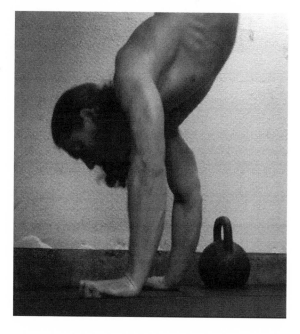

Workout A
Upper body pushing exercise
Upper body pulling exercise

Workout B
Lower body squat exercise
Ab exercise

Each workout, both A and B can then be done two or three times per week in alternating fashion.

What about…?

What about grip? What about bridging? What about ABC or XYZ?

This template is not meant to cover ALL bases, but just the basics. There are several things that can be added into it such as bridging (gymnast and wrestlers), grip work, other tools and more.

These different exercises can be done before or after the main workout. They can also be mixed into the circuit.

More conditioning can be added with the addition of burpees, jump rope or other methods as well.

While we are focused on bodyweight training here, recognize that this same template works outside of it, with any training tool.

And while we're at it I might add that bodyweight training has a disadvantage in that there is no lower body pulling exercise. Think deadlift or kettlebell swing. This is a "gap" that occurs with bodyweight training that can be remedied by using other tools. Do you absolutely need it? No, not unless your goals involve doing those moves specifically. But if you do want ultimate well-rounded athleticism and strength it's good to have in there.

There are infinite ways you could change up this basic workout plan, but I wanted to be sure that I gave you something to get started with.

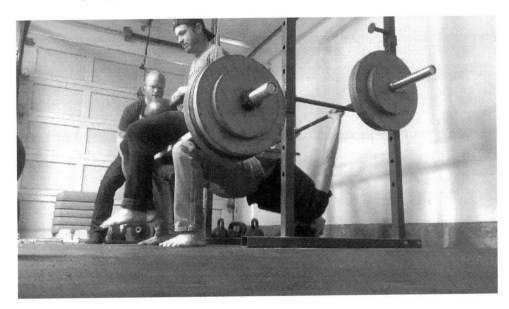

More Examples

I'm providing a few more examples of sticking exercises, set and reps into the template in order to clear up any misunderstandings as well as bring up some additional points.

Pike Press x 5 x 10
Weighted Pullup x 3 x 5
Pistol Squat x 10 x 2 L/R
Full Hanging Knee Raise x 5 x 10
(L/R means left and right, in this case 10 sets of 2 for each leg.)

Notice that in this example you're not doing the same number of sets of each exercise. Some of the exercises are with harder progressions than others, and thus, there are fewer reps per set. In this example, a person may just have achieved pistol squats and is forced to do low rep sets but can "practice" lots of them by doing more sets.

What follows are an example of three workouts that could be done in a week. The first is higher volume but easier exercises. The last is higher intensity but light on volume. The middle one is in the middle.

Workout A (Week 1)
Pushup x 6 x 20
Inverted Row x 6 x 20
Basic Squat x 6 x 40
V-ups x 6 x 20

Workout B (Week 1)
Dive Bomber Pushups x 4 x 8
Chin-ups x 4 x 6
Box Jump Squats x 4 x 10
Hanging Leg Raises 90 Degrees x 4 x 6

Workout C (Week 1)
Handstand pushups x 5 x 3
Muscle Up x 5 x 2
Pistol Squats x 5 x 3 L/R
Hanging Leg Raises 180 Degrees x 5 x 3

That is one week of workouts. Then you could work on the same variations the next week, but you would aim to do a little more. For instance:

Workout A (Week 2)
Pushup x 7 x 20
Inverted Row x 7 x 20
Basic Squat x 7 x 40
V-ups x 7 x 20

Workout B (Week 2)
Dive Bomber Pushups x 4 x 10
Chin-ups x 4 x 7
Box Jump Squats x 4 x 12
Hanging Leg Raises 90 Degrees x 4 x 8

Workout C (Week 1)
Handstand pushups x 6 x 3
Muscle Up x 6 x 2
Pistol Squats x 6 x 3 L/R
Hanging Leg Raises 180 Degrees x 6 x 3

Notice that there was a mix in progressions here. Some things were progressed by adding another set in Workouts A and C. Some things were progressed by adding more reps in Workout B.

Let's say you continue on this for a number of weeks and then we'll just take workout A as an example. If you continued in it, adding a set each week you would arrive at:

Workout A (Week 5)
Pushup x 10 x 20
Inverted Row x 10 x 20
Basic Squat x 10 x 40
V-ups x 10 x 20

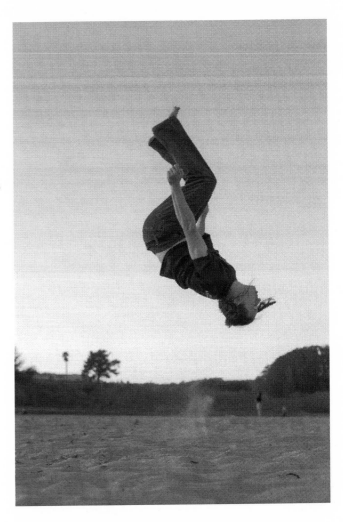

That's a lot of volume and notice we are at the top end of the recommended set and reps. At this point your next jump would be in difficulty of the exercises, and in doing so you're going to drop down in volume, which could be in sets, reps or both.

Workout A (Week 6)
Decline Pushups x 5 x 15
Inverted Row Straight Legs x 5 x 15
Side to Side Squat x 5 x 30
Hanging Knee Raise 90 Degrees x 5 x 12

That's a quick lesson in progression and how you will progress in using this template.

The main thing is to start using it as that is the only way to build the experience into your body. You'll discover much along the way as you proceed along your bodyweight journey.

About the Author

Born without genetic gifts, a weak and scrawny Logan Christopher sought out the best training information in his pursuit of super strength, mind power and radiant health. Nowadays, he's known for his famous feats of pulling an 8,800 lb. firetruck by his hair, juggling flaming kettlebells, and supporting half a ton in the wrestler's bridge. Called the "Physical Culture Renaissance Man" his typical workouts might include backflips, freestanding handstand pushups, tearing phonebooks in half, bending steel, deadlifting a heavy barbell, or lifting rocks overhead.

Far from being all brawn and no brain Logan has sought optimal performance with mental training and sports psychology which he has explored in depth, becoming an NLP Trainer, certified hypnotist, EFT practitioner and more. That's also how he got started in the field of health and nutrition which inevitably led to Chinese, Ayurvedic and Western herbalism.

His personal philosophy is to bring together the best movement skill, health information, and mental training to achieve peak performance. He is the author of many books and video programs to help people increase their strength, skills, health and mental performance. Discover how you too can become super strong, both mentally and physically, at www.LegendaryStrength.com and find the superior herbs to support all aspects of your performance at www.LostEmpireHerbs.com.

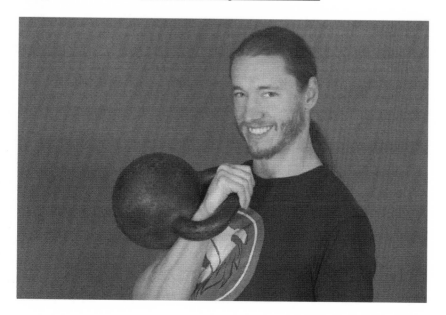

Other Books by Logan Christopher

- The Master Keys to Strength and Fitness
- Deceptive Strength
- The Indestructible Body
- Practicing Strength and Movement: How to Gain Any Skill FASTER!
- The Ultimate Guide to Handstand Pushups
- The Ultimate Guide to Pullups and Chin-ups
- The Ultimate Guide to Bodyweight Ab Exercises
- The Ultimate Guide to Bodyweight Conditioning
- Secrets of the Handstand
- Learn How to Back Flip in 31 Days
- 101 Simple Steps to Radiant Health
- 101 Advanced Steps to Radiant Health
- Upgrade Your Breath
- Upgrade Your Testosterone
- Upgrade Your Growth Hormone
- Berzerker: Psyching Up for Strength and Sports
- Mental Muscle

**For a full up-to-date list of titles plus and videos and more
from Logan Christopher go to:
www.LegendaryStrength.com/books-videos/**

"Get Stronger... Move Better... Become Healthier... Unleash Your Mind Power... Every Single Month"

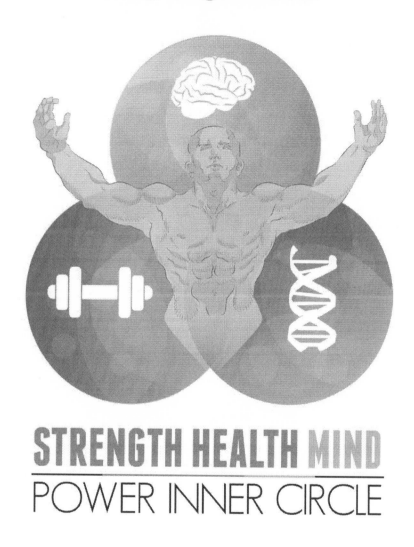

STRENGTH HEALTH MIND
POWER INNER CIRCLE

- Monthly Newsletter on Achieving Peak Health & Performance
- Access to Coaching from Logan Christopher
- Private Community of Members
- Free Bonuses and Videos
- And Much More

www.StrengthHealthMindPower.com

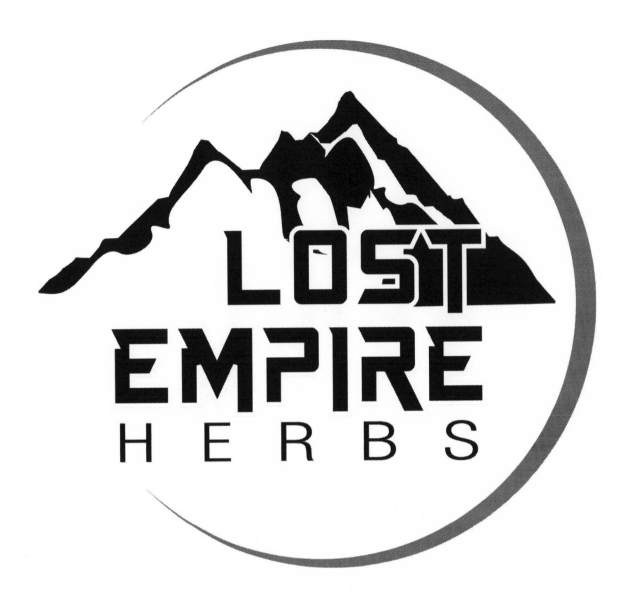

Superior Herbs for All Your Performance Needs

- Potent Herbal Extracts Where You Feel a Difference in Your Health and Performance
- Hormones, Athletics, Cognitive Performance and More
- 100% All Natural with No Fillers or Additives
- Guaranteed to Work…Or Your Money Back

www.LostEmpireHerbs.com

Made in the USA
Middletown, DE
01 November 2018